thefacts

D0100972

Prenatal tests and ultrasound

ELIZABETH CRABTREE BURTON

Chief Sonographer, Ultrasound,
Millburn Ob/Gyn Associates, New Jersey, USA

RICHARD L. LUCIANI

Physician Director, Millburn Ob/Gyn Associates,
New Jersey, USA
Attending Physician at St Barnabas Medical Center,
Livingston, New Jersey, and Overlook Hospital, Summit,
New Jersey, USA

OXFORD
UNIVERSITY PRESS

OXFORD
UNIVERSITY PRESS

Great Clarendon Street, Oxford OX2 6DP

Oxford University Press is a department of the University of Oxford.
It furthers the University's objective of excellence in research, scholarship,
and education by publishing worldwide in

Oxford New York

Auckland Cape Town Dar es Salaam Hong Kong Karachi
Kuala Lumpur Madrid Melbourne Mexico City Nairobi
New Delhi Shanghai Taipei Toronto

With offices in

Argentina Austria Brazil Chile Czech Republic France Greece
Guatemala Hungary Italy Japan Poland Portugal Singapore
South Korea Switzerland Thailand Turkey Ukraine Vietnam

Oxford is a registered trade mark of Oxford University Press
in the UK and in certain other countries

Published in the United States
by Oxford University Press Inc., New York

British Library Cataloguing in Publication Data

Data available

Library of Congress Cataloging in Publication Data

Data available

ISBN 978-0-19-959930-1

10 9 8 7 6 5 4 3 2 1

Typeset in Plantin by Cenveo, Bangalore, India
Printed in Great Britain
on acid-free paper by
Ashford Colour Press Ltd, Gosport, Hampshire

Preface

You've discovered that you are pregnant, or someone you care about is pregnant. After that initial rush of excitement, you start to have a lot of questions. Is the baby healthy? Is he or she growing well? From the moment a woman suspects that she is pregnant, the testing begins, and so do the questions. Can she trust the home pregnancy test kits? When is it time to go to the doctor or midwife? After coming to terms with the fact that pregnancy has occurred, the next step is often to worry about whether everything is progressing normally. From the first medical visit to the time of birth, every appointment is likely to involve some sort of testing, whether it is as simple as weight, urine, and blood pressure, or more complicated, involving blood tests, genetic screening, and ultrasounds. Pregnancy is **not** a disease, yet all the testing associated with it can provoke a lot of anxiety and confusion for families. There are plenty of pregnancy-related sources explaining all the changes and physical symptoms of pregnancy, but not many provide a clear explanation of all the prenatal tests in one source. With this book, women will find a clear timeline and explanation of all the tests they can expect to be offered at each stage of pregnancy, and how and why they are performed. It is important to note that this book is intended to explain the types of tests you are likely to encounter in most locations, but some of the tests we discuss may or may not be offered routinely in every country, medical practice, or locale. This book is not intended to offer medical advice or be a substitute for good antenatal care. Not every test that we discuss in this book is appropriate for every person. There will be variations in practice depending on where you live, your medical history, and your family history. Your health care provider will know which of these many tests are appropriate for **your** specific situation, and when the optimal time arises for administering them.

Testing can be broadly divided into two categories. In one section, we will address the many tests that assess the general health of the mother. Evaluating the mother is important to ensure that her health status is not being adversely affected by her pregnancy, and that she is in optimal condition to nurture the developing fetus. In other sections, we will address screening and testing of the fetus. This type of testing is offered because even if the mother is in peak physical condition, with no family history of problems, the baby may still suffer from chromosomal, genetic, or anatomical abnormalities. Families need to understand that there are different testing options available to screen for fetuses which may be genetically or physically abnormal, and there is a difference between *screening* tests and *diagnostic* tests. Screening tests carry no risk to the fetus or mother, but may give a falsely positive or falsely negative result. These tests carry the potential to induce a lot of anxiety that the baby may be abnormal when, in fact, there are no problems at all. Receiving an abnormal result on a screening test requires a decision about whether or not to put the pregnancy at risk with a more invasive test. Diagnostic testing requires thoughtful consideration, because there is a small risk that performing the test can cause a miscarriage, but the results are 100% accurate. An abnormal result on this type of test allows for termination of the pregnancy, if that is an option and a parental choice. If not, it allows parents to make the proper preparations for birth and caring for a child with an impairment. Because people have very different beliefs and attitudes about raising a child with a disability, not all types of testing are appropriate for every family. This book aims to be an informational source which clarifies the pros and cons of each type of test, empowering parents to choose the testing options with which they are most comfortable.

With so many routine available tests, it is no wonder that parents become confused about which tests that they can **opt** to have versus those that they **should** have. For example, older mothers may say 'I'm going to be 38 so I have to get an amniocentesis'. It's very important that parents understand that they don't **have** to have an amniocentesis or many of the other screening tests that are offered. This is not your doctor or midwife's pregnancy, it is yours. Your doctor or midwife certainly wouldn't want to perform a test on you that has a risk of miscarriage unless you and your partner understand the risks and are willing to accept the possibility of losing the pregnancy. There is a difference between a test being *recommended* for you versus being *offered* to you. Your provider will definitely *recommend* that you have your urine and your blood pressure checked, etc. (tests described in Chapter 5). By doing those types of tests, your provider is able to monitor and protect your health which in turn ensures the best possible environment for the fetus to develop, grow, and have a successful birth. Should the tests show something to be concerned about, your provider can take steps to manage or even avoid scenarios that might otherwise result in a poor outcome for the mother or baby.

This is very different than testing to ensure that the fetus itself is 'normal.' This type of screening or testing is *offered* to you, you have the choice to take advantage of it or not. It is your provider's job to let you know what types of testing are available, including offering additional testing that may be appropriate if you are at high risk for an abnormal baby for any reason. He or she is not going to think you are a bad person or irresponsible parent for choosing to test or not to test. You may be the type of person who wants every test available to find out if your baby has a problem, even if you are low risk. Or, you may feel that you would never terminate a pregnancy with abnormalities and you would prefer to enjoy the nine months uncomplicated by potentially worrisome test results. Or you may be somewhere in between. Your care provider almost certainly has seen the full spectrum of different attitudes and beliefs and is there to guide you to the proper personal choice. By learning about the tests that are available, you can accept the level of testing which is appropriate for you.

This book also intends to explain ultrasound imaging, which has become an iconic part of being pregnant and is arguably one of the most powerful tools in prenatal testing practice. The ultrasound experience can certainly be one of the highlights of a pregnancy. Women can hardly get out of the door without their mobile phones ringing with calls from excited grandparents, friends, and siblings, all of whom look forward to seeing the pictures. However, many people, especially first time parents, have no idea what actually happens during their ultrasounds or how many examinations are performed in an average pregnancy, and would like to know more about what providers are looking for when we are taking all those pictures. Women and their partners often present with many good questions (and some misconceptions) about their examination such as:

◈ Is ultrasound safe?

◈ How does ultrasound get a picture?

◈ Does the baby have a good heartbeat?

◈ How do you determine the sex?

◈ Which do I believe, my provider's due date or the ultrasound due date?

◈ How can I be sure there's only one baby in there?

◈ Are 3D/4D scans better?

This book is designed to answer all these questions and more. The information presented here will help to guide pregnant women and their partners and relatives through the sometimes overwhelming battery of testing that often begins from the moment a pregnancy is suspected and applies to most normal, average pregnancies. The good news is that the vast majority of pregnancies are relatively uneventful and the end result is a beautiful, healthy newborn. Occasionally, some pregnancies are not routine or are considered high risk for a multitude of different reasons. This book is not intended to focus on all the things that can go wrong, nor can it offer advice on further tests or treatments. The possible complications are too many and too individual to be adequately addressed in this or any single book. Should your routine testing uncover something that requires additional tests or medical management, your midwife or doctor is best suited to discuss this with you, and to offer resources and referrals based on your personal circumstances. A list of websites and resources is included at the end of the book, and can be referred to for further information.

As a final note, this book has been carefully written with the intent that it be a useful resource for an international audience. Standards of care in each country do differ, so some of the tests offered routinely in the United States may not be considered routine in the United Kingdom or other countries and vice versa. We have tried to cover all tests that you might encounter no matter where you live. Medical as well as some general terminology between the countries also differs, and we have made an effort to appeal to all audiences, but it is likely that there will be some occasional unfamiliarity with terms. We have included a glossary to be referred to when needed. Finally, there is a great variety of titles for the types of practitioners who are responsible for caring for women during a pregnancy such as nurse practitioners, midwives, physician assistants, doctors and obstetricians. To be as general as possible, we will use the term 'provider' or 'care provider' to include all of these important roles.

Contents

Glossary of terms

Abortion: Interruption of pregnancy. This can be voluntarily induced or spontaneous. A spontaneous abortion is an unintended failure of the pregnancy to progress and subsequent natural loss of the products of conception. A voluntarily induced abortion is also known as pregnancy termination.

AFP/alpha-fetoprotein: Protein produced by the fetus that can be found in the maternal blood. Elevated levels can indicate an open defect of the spine, head, or abdomen in the fetus. Decreased levels can signal Down's syndrome.

Amniotic fluid: The fluid that surrounds the fetus within the amniotic sac.

Amniocentesis: Passage of a needle into the amniotic sac to take a sample of the amniotic fluid for testing, usually performed around 16 weeks. Amniocentesis can also be performed later in the pregnancy to assess fetal lung maturity.

Anomaly: Abnormality.

Antenatal: The time before birth, also known as 'prenatal.'

Blighted ovum: A failed pregnancy where there is a gestational sac and early placental tissue growing, but an embryo failed to develop. This is the most common type of miscarriage. The lack of a viable (live) pregnancy may be 'missed' by the body for many weeks, requiring that a surgical procedure be performed to remove the products of conception.

Breech: Presentation of the fetus with the head up and rump or feet at the cervix.

Cervix: Narrow lower part of the uterus which acts as a gateway between the uterus and the vagina.

Chromosomes: A long molecule of DNA and associated amino acids that carry genes and the hereditary information of an organism. Humans should have 23 matched pairs.

Chorionic villi: Branching finger-like projections of early placental tissue which develop to grow into a fully functioning placenta.

Chorionic villus sampling (CVS): Procedure to obtain a sampling of the chorionic villi (early placental tissue), which contains the fetal chromosomes that can be analyzed and tested to assess the structure and number of chromosomes. In some cases, additional testing can be done to detect specific inherited diseases.

Conception: Moment where sperm meets egg and cell division begins. Usually occurs approximately 2 weeks from the first day of the last menstrual period (LMP).

Crown-rump length: Measurement of the embryo from end to end in early pregnancy, used to date the gestation age.

Corpus luteal cyst: Cyst on the ovary that is normally created during ovulation. After the egg has been released, the area where the egg was shed from becomes the 'corpus luteum' and secretes estrogens and progesterone to prepare the uterine lining for implantation and pregnancy. It usually disappears on its own after 12 weeks.

CVS/Chorionic villus sampling: Procedure to obtain chorionic villi (developing placental cells) in order to analyze the fetal chromosomes. The procedure can be performed transabdominally (via the abdomen) or transvaginally (via the cervix) between 10.5 and 13 weeks.

Cytogenetics: Study of the structure and function of hereditary cells, specifically the chromosomes.

D&C/Dilatation and curettage: Surgical procedure to remove the products of pregnancy using suction, usually performed before 13 weeks.

D&E/Dilatation and evacuation: Surgical procedure to remove the products of pregnancy with specialized instruments and suction, usually performed after 13 weeks.

Doppler (in the case of fetal heart detection): The use of sound waves to detect motion in order to create an audible sound of blood flowing in arteries, veins, and the heart.

Down's syndrome: An extra chromosome at the 21st pair, known as trisomy 21, resulting in moderate to severe mental retardation, upward slanting eyes, usually with epicanthic folds, a broad short skull, broad hands with short fingers, and decreased muscle tone.

Ectopic pregnancy: Pregnancy that has implanted outside of the uterus.

EDD: Estimated date of delivery/birth. Also known as the 'estimated due date', which is 40 weeks from the first day of the last menstrual period (LMP) or 38 weeks from conception, based on a 28 day menstrual cycle.

Embryo: Term for developing human from conception to approximately 8 weeks post-conception or 10 weeks from the first day of the last menstrual period (LMP).

False negative: Incorrect test result where the test showed no sign of abnormality, yet an abnormality is present.

False positive: Incorrect test result where the test is positive for high risk of an abnormality to be present, when in fact no abnormality exists.

Fetus: Term for developing human once it has progressed beyond the embryo stage, from 8 weeks after conception (approximately 10 weeks from the LMP) until birth.

Fibroid: Benign thickening or tumour of the uterine muscle, also called a fibromyoma or leiomyoma.

FISH Testing/Flourescent *in situ* hybridization: Specialized lab technique allowing for the rapid turnaround of chromosomal studies: only counts chromosomes looking for trisomy 13, 18, 21, and X/Y chromosomes. Results can be available within 48 to 72 hours.

Fraternal twins: Also known as non-identical twins. Conceived from two separate fertilized eggs, each one always has its own placenta and amniotic sac.

Fundus: Top of the uterus.

Genes: A region of DNA that controls a hereditary characteristic. It usually corresponds to a sequence used in the production of a specific protein or RNA.

Genetic counsellor: Medical professional who is an expert in genetic abnormalities and inheritability of diseases.

Geneticist: Physician specializing in inherited diseases.

Gestational age: Age of a pregnancy based on the weeks since the first day of the last menstrual period (LMP).

Gestational sac: The rounded sac in the uterus, surrounded by early placental tissue where the embryo develops. This will grow into the amniotic sac or cavity.

Gestational diabetes: Condition in pregnancy where a previously non-diabetic woman develops high blood sugar. Adjustments in diet may control the condition, but it may be necessary to treat with medications, including insulin. Gestational diabetes will disappear after the birth of the baby.

Hypertension: High blood pressure.

hCG/Human chorionic gonadotropin: pregnancy hormone produced by the developing placenta that can be found in the blood or urine to diagnose pregnancy.

Identical twins: Conceived from a single egg and sperm that divides into two individual embryos. Whether or not they each have their own placenta or amniotic sac depends on how early the fertilized egg splits. Fertilized eggs that split later can share a placenta, sac, or even be conjoined.

Karyotype: A picture of chromosomes arranged and analyzed according to number, size, and form.

LMP/Last menstrual period: Used to date the pregnancy, done by counting from the first day of the last menstrual menstruation.

Missed abortion: Failed pregnancy with or without a non-viable (demised) embryo that has not yet spontaneously been expelled from the uterus. A surgical abortion may be necessary to remove the products of conception.

Miscarriage: Unintended loss of a pregnancy, either spontaneously where it passes on its own, or facilitated by a surgical procdure such as a D&C or D&E.

Neonate: Newborn.

Non-identical Twins: Also known as fraternal twins. Conceived from two separate fertilized eggs, each one always has its own placenta and amniotic sac.

Nuchal translucency: Thin pocket of fluid that lies under the skin behind the fetal neck, best observed and measured between 10.5 and 13 weeks.

A thicker-than-expected measurement can indicate a chromosomal or structural problem.

Oligohydramnios: Decreased amniotic fluid volume.

Ovulation: Process by which a ripe egg is expelled from the ovary. The expulsion of the egg (ovulation) usually occurs around 14 days after the first day of the last menstrual period (LMP).

Placenta: An organ that develops after conception to connect the fetus with the uterine wall and maternal blood supply, allows for the exchange of oxygen, nutrients, and waste.

Placenta praevia: Condition where the placenta implants directly above the cervix. In these cases, once the cervix starts to dilate, severe hemorrhaging can occur with potential for fetal and even maternal death. If there is a placenta previa, the baby will need to be delivered a few weeks early via cesarean section.

Polyhydramnios: Increased amniotic fluid volume.

Pre-eclampsia: Serious condition that can occur anytime in the second half of pregnancy where there is an increase in blood pressure, fluid retention, and protein in the urine. The woman may also experience headaches and abdominal pain. It impacts the fetus negatively, causing decreased blow flow through the placenta as well as other potential problems. If the condition progresses, it can lead to eclampsia which causes severe toxicity, convulsions, and even death.

Pregnancy termination: Voluntarily induced abortion.

Prenatal: Existing or ocurring before birth, also known as 'antenatal'.

Progesterone: hormone in pregnancy initially secreted by corpus luteal cyst in the ovary to support the early developing pregnancy.

Prophylactic: Preventative

Rhesus disease: see Rh Incompatabililty.

Rh factor: A genetically determined protein in the blood that some people have and others don't. Rh positive indicates those with the protein, Rh negative indicates those without the protein.

Rh Incompatibility: If a fetus is Rh Positive but the mother is Rh negative, a serious immunogenic reaction can occur in which the mother produces antibodies that cross the placenta and attack the red blood cells of the fetus causing severe, often life-threatening fetal anemia—also called Rhesus disease.

Serum testing: testing done on a maternal blood sample.

Soft marker: Anatomical variations that are not abnormal or cause problems in the fetus, but have been loosely correlated to be a possible flag for Down's syndrome or other chromosomal abnormality.

Transducer: Device that emits ultrasound waves that are transmitted into human tissue. Also called an ultrasound probe, different types include transabdominal or transvaginal.

Trisomy: An abnormality of chromosomes where an additional chromosome is present. Chromosomes should come in 23 pairs, an additional chromosome at any of the pairs is known as a trisomy. The three most common are Trisomy 21 (Down Syndrome), Trisomy 18 (Edward Syndrome), and Trisomy 13 (Patau Syndrome).

Trimester: The entire pregnancy is divided into three trimesters; 1st trimester is approximately from weeks 0–12, 2nd trimester is approximately weeks 13–28, and the 3rd trimester is approximately weeks 29–40.

Ultrasound: The use of high frequency sound waves sent into the body to create an image of internal organ structures.

Vertex: Head-first presentation of the fetus, also called 'cephalic'.

Yolk sac: Membranous sac attached to the early developing embryo that supplies nutrients. It becomes obsolete by approximately 12 weeks when the placenta becomes fully functioning. The yolk sac is visible on ultrasound by approximately 5.5 menstrual weeks, even before the embryo is visible.

1

Diagnosing pregnancy

➔ Key points

♦ Pregnancy tests detect the hormone human chorionic gonadotropin (hCG). This hormone is secreted during pregnancy by the developing placenta and is detectable in urine and blood.

♦ Using current tests, hCG can be detected in urine as early as 10 to 12 days after conception. At this stage, these tests are 95–98% accurate if the result is positive.

♦ In the blood, hCG can be detected as soon as 7 or 8 days after conception, and is a highly accurate way of determining whether implantation of the fertilized egg has occurred. In cases where problems are suspected, repeated blood tests can help to predict whether or not the pregnancy is progressing normally.

♦ Progesterone is another hormone detectable in the blood that can be used to assess the viability of a pregnancy. It is secreted by a part of the ovary (known as a corpus luteum) following ovulation.

For many women, pregnancy is suspected due to a missed period. However, this is not always a reliable indicator that a woman is in fact pregnant. The diagnosis of pregnancy is one that stirs up the most intense of emotions in women, from a feeling of total joy and exhilaration to feelings of anxiety or helplessness. It often prompts lifestyle changes, and it is therefore extremely important to establish this diagnosis in a timely and accurate way. The most common method of diagnosing pregnancy is via a simple urine test, which can be bought without a prescription at most pharmacies. Pregnancy hormones can also be detected in the blood, although blood tests are not usually necessary unless there is spotting, bleeding, or other concerns. In this chapter, we will explain how these tests work and review their accuracy.

Pregnancy tests detect the 'pregnancy' hormone, called human chorionic gonadotropin (hCG). You will often hear your healthcare provider refer to the pregnancy test as the 'beta hCG' test. This is because the hormone hCG is a large protein molecule, composed of alpha and beta subunits. The alpha subunit is very similar to those of several other hormones, including follicle stimulating hormone (FSH) and thyrotropin (thyroid hormone). However, the beta subunit of hCG is different, making it easy to detect and much more specific to pregnancy. This beta hCG subunit becomes detectable in the mother's urine and blood soon after conception.

Measurement of the hCG hormone level in blood or urine offers the quickest and most accurate result for establishing whether a woman is pregnant. However, hCG is released by the developing placenta after implantation of the egg has occurred, not by the developing fetus. Therefore, the hCG test does not detect the presence of a live embryo (also known as a 'viable' pregnancy); it only reflects the presence of early placental cells.

Urine pregnancy test

Initially, you may choose to do a home urine pregnancy test. These tests are extremely convenient, inexpensive, and may be purchased at most pharmacies and grocery stores without the need for a doctor's prescription. The accuracy rate of these urine pregnancy tests approaches 95% to 98%, and can sometimes detect pregnancy as early as a day or two before the next period is due. Of extreme importance is the fact that a positive urine test is much more likely to be correct than a negative one. If the test is negative, it doesn't necessarily mean you aren't pregnant: it may be too soon for the hormone to be detected. Trying again in a few days may yield a positive result.

Blood pregnancy test

Modern urine tests are so accurate that it is not usually necessary to perform blood tests except in specific cases. If you have spotting, severe pain, or other unusual symptoms, your healthcare provider may decide to send you for a blood test and an early ultrasound scan (described in Chapter 7). The blood test can measure the numerical level of hCG. This test is more sensitive than the urine test, and only rarely gives a false negative result.

In over 95% of pregnant women, hCG is detectable in the maternal blood from 8 to 10 days after conception. The amount of beta hCG in the blood should double every 2 to 3 days in the early stages of pregnancy, making it an useful hormone for establishing pregnancy viability (in other words, the presence of a live embryo) and for detecting abnormal gestations such as a blighted ovum or ectopic pregnancy. A blighted ovum (also known as a missed abortion) happens when the implantation of the fertilized egg occurs and a gestational sac starts to grow, but an embryo fails to develop. The placental tissue will remain in the uterus and continue to grow, but the gestational sac is empty. Ectopic pregnancies are pregnancies that implant and grow outside of the uterus which can have serious consequences if not detected early. When your healthcare provider is unsure of the viability or location of your pregnancy, monitoring the rise of the beta hCG levels in the blood can be extremely helpful.

Progesterone

Another important hormone utilized in monitoring a viable versus non-viable pregnancy is called progesterone. This hormone is produced by a normal cystic structure on the surface of the ovary known as the corpus luteum. A viable (live) pregnancy is likely if the serum progesterone level is greater than 25 ng/ml. If the level is less than 5 ng/ml, there is a high suspicion that the pregnancy is not going to progress. If the blood test is between 5 and 25 ng/ml, this suggests you should probably be evaluated with further diagnostic testing, including an ultrasound scan.

What happens next? Once you have tested positive for pregnancy, it is time to contact your clinic or care provider to set up your first prenatal appointment. At this first appointment, you will often be offered a variety of tests to check your health and assess your genetic risks. Your provider will explain the timeline of the various tests being offered to you, leaving you with a lot of decisions to make in the coming weeks. The following chapters will help you to make sense of these tests, so you can understand what is being offered and why, allowing you to make informed decisions about what is right for you.

2

Genetic screening of the parents

➡ Key points

⬩ At an early prenatal visit, family history and ethnicity will be discussed in detail with the care provider. Based on this information, it is possible to screen the mother's blood for diseases of which her child may be at higher risk. Some common examples are cystic fibrosis, thalassemia, and sickle cell anaemia.

⬩ Genes are codes in our body, contained within DNA, that determine our physical characteristics and body chemistry. Mistakes or mutations within genes can cause a host of debilitating or even fatal inherited diseases.

⬩ Screening the parents for inherited genetic diseases is **not the same** as screening the fetus for Down's syndrome or other chromosomal problems. This type of testing is fully discussed in the next chapter.

⬩ Even if no one in either parent's family history has actually suffered from an inherited disease, it is still possible that they carry an affected gene. If both parents have the same recessive mutation, there is a 25% chance that their child will suffer from the disease.

⬩ If there is a strong family history of a particular disease, or if both parents are found to be carriers for a gene mutation, additional testing can be performed on the fetus to determine whether it is affected by the disease.

.ne previous chapter we discussed diagnosing pregnancy. Once a pregnancy nas been confirmed, a comprehensive assessment by your doctor and/or midwife will follow. You will be asked to provide detailed family and personal medical histories. Current technology offers many new possibilities for disease detection, and this includes looking for genetic predispositions for inherited diseases. Hundreds of tests of blood or tissue are now available for identifying genes that may predispose us or our offspring to develop a specific disease. You can expect to be advised on the many types of tests that are offered, and which are recommended based on your history. If your ethnicity or history indicate that you may be at higher risk for a specific disease, your provider can request special testing in the batch of initial prenatal blood tests.

Any test that is offered during the pregnancy must only be done with the express consent of the pregnant woman, after a full explanation from the provider of the advantages and disadvantages of each test. If you do not understand or are uncomfortable with the tests that are being offered, you should have an open and honest discussion with your provider about your concerns.

Prenatal genetic screening is now available to those couples who wish to improve their chances of carrying a genetically normal infant to term. There are many rare but very serious diseases that parents can unwittingly pass on to their children. Some examples are sickle cell anaemia, cystic fibrosis, Gaucher's disease, and spinal muscular atrophy. Affected children can appear normal at birth, but symptoms may appear in the first years or even months of life. Diagnosis of an inherited disease is a cause of shock and dismay to families. In the past, parents had very little chance of knowing that they were carriers of these diseases until they manifested in their children. Today, developments in DNA sequencing and analysis mean that your carrier status for some of these diseases can be determined in early pregnancy, or before.

Screening for gene defects vs. chromosomal abnormalities

Screening the mother's blood for the presence of gene mutations is **not** the same as screening the fetus for abnormalities. Genetic screening of the parents establishes their potential risk of passing inherited diseases on to their children. In contrast, screening of the fetus (explained in Chapter 3) is done to look for an abnormal number of chromosomes, such as occurs with Down's syndrome, or abnormalities in chromosome shape and structure. Most of the time, Down's syndrome and similar chromosomal abnormalities occur in isolation and are not inherited from either parent.

Our DNA, genes and chromosomes

DNA: A very long molecule containing a code written in four building blocks or 'letters,' which are 'read' by the cell and which control the development of all the body's structures and functions.

Gene: A stretch of DNA encoding a particular function, e.g. eye pigment, and forming <u>part</u> of a chromosome, by which inherited characteristics are transmitted from parent to offspring.

Chromosome: A microscopic rod-shaped structure that appears in the cell during cell division, which consists of a long, looped string of DNA containing multiple genes.

What is carrier status?

By testing a blood sample from the mother, it is possible to determine whether or not she is carrying a gene associated with a specific disease. Genes are the chemical 'instructions' in the cells of our body that determine and map out who we actually are. Genes can be normal or they can mutate to become abnormal. If a gene is mutated, it may cause a disorder in the body's structure or chemistry to occur, which can lead to the development of a disease.

Typical Jewish heritage panel

- Tay-Sachs

- Canavan disease

- Familial dysautonomia

- Bloom syndrome

- Gaucher's disease

- Fanconi anaemia

- Mucolipidosis type IV

- Fanconi anaemia

- Niemann-Pick type A

We have two copies of each human gene (except for some genes specific to men), and we inherit one copy from each parent. Some problems can arise when only one copy is faulty; these are known as **autosomal dominant** diseases. If either the mother or father has a dominant mutation, they will be affected by the disease, and they have a 50% chance of passing it on to their offspring.

Many genetic diseases require two faulty copies of a gene to be present before symptoms occur, however. In these instances, carriers of a single mutated gene will not normally be affected by the disease which the gene is known to cause, but they can pass that gene on to their offspring. These conditions, where the child must inherit the same gene mutation from **each** parent for disease to occur, are called **autosomal recessive** diseases. If both parents are found to be carriers of the same mutated gene, there is a 25% chance that their child will suffer from the disease. Therefore, if the mother tests positive in the initial screening for a specific autosomal recessive gene defect, it will be necessary to bring in the father for testing. Since most genetic abnormalities are rare, the father is likely to test negative for the same mutation. There is then no cause for concern; although the child may carry the mutation, they will not be affected by disease. On the other hand, if the father is found to be a carrier too, further testing with chorionic villus sampling (CVS) or amniocentesis can be offered to determine whether the fetus has the disease (see Chapter 4).

Finally, some genetic disorders are caused by mutations in genes located within the sex chromosomes, X and Y. Baby boys and girls will therefore have different levels of risk for these diseases, if their parents are carriers. One example is haemophilia, a blood-clotting disorder, which is carried on the X chromosome. With two X chromosomes, girls are less likely to be affected as they would have to inherit a damaged X from both parents to have the disease. Boys have only one X chromosome; if this carries the haemophilia mutation they will develop the disease. Your family medical history will be taken into account by your provider in determining whether your fetus is at risk of sex-chromosome linked diseases.

Role of ethnicity and disease

Certain diseases occur much more often in some ethnic groups than in others. By looking at affected individuals within these targeted ethnic groups, scientists are able to find and identify the most common gene mutations linked to each disease. The standard screening tests search only for these more common mutations. Different mutations may occur, so it is possible that someone could still be a disease carrier, but test negative for the most common gene defects. Fortunately, these sorts of mutations are very rare.

Your provider will know the appropriate tests to order based on your individual family history and ethnicity. For example, if you are Caucasian, you might be tested for the mutations most commonly associated with cystic fibrosis, since 1 in 29 Caucasians are cystic fibrosis carriers. If you are of Ashkenazi (European) Jewish descent, there is an entire panel of diseases that tend to occur within that ethnic group, for which routine testing may be done (see box). The frequency of carrier status for these diseases in Ashkenazi Jews ranges from 1 in 30 for Tay-Sachs disease, to 1 in 100 for Bloom syndrome.

Carrier status vs. presence of disease

If a woman is at high risk of passing on a specific disease based on family history, or if both parents are found during screening to be carriers of a known recessive gene mutation, further testing can be done during the pregnancy to determine whether the fetus is affected by the disease. Even if both parents are carriers of a recessive mutation linked to a disease, it is still possible to have a healthy child. As described above, there is only approximately a 1 in 4 or 25% chance of the fetus having two mutated copies of the affected gene. CVS or amniocentesis can be performed to obtain a sample of fetal tissue, which can then be analyzed to diagnose the presence or absence of a specific disease. A full discussion of CVS, amniocentesis, and the results can be found in Chapter 4.

Pre-pregnancy screening

Genetic screening can be performed on the mother's blood before pregnancy occurs; this is also known as pre-conception testing. Because of the financial cost, it is usually only done by parents-to-be when there is a higher than average risk of having a baby with a specific disease, either due to a strong family history or an unusually high incidence within their particular ethnic group. If the potential parents are indeed found to be carriers, after they conceive they can seek early diagnosis with CVS, which can be done before the end of the first trimester.

Another option is to undergo pre-implantation testing, although this method is expensive and requires that the parents conceive via in-vitro fertilization (IVF). In addition, the technologies and expertise required are only available in the most advanced specialist centres. In these cases, the mother's eggs are surgically harvested and fertilized with the father's sperm in the laboratory. Once the cells have divided a few times, a single cell from each resulting embryo can be removed and tested for the disease-causing mutation. An embryo, or embryos, without the mutation are then selectively transferred into the uterus.

3

Genetic screening of the fetus

⊃ Key points

◆ Genetic screening is done by taking a blood sample from the mother, posing no harm to the fetus.

◆ Genetic screening differs from genetic testing: screening only tells you that there MAY be a problem with the fetus. Genetic testing will diagnose if there really IS a problem with the fetus.

◆ Genetic screening gives a numerical risk assessment of the likelihood that your baby could be abnormal. You are considered 'high risk' if your odds are found to be greater than around 1 in 200 to 1 in 300.

◆ Genetic screening will miss a small percentage of abnormal babies.

◆ There are many more false positives (meaning you are told you are at high risk but your baby is actually normal) than true positives.

◆ Genetic screening is optional. It is important to consider in advance whether or not you want to know if you are at higher risk.

◆ There are many different varieties of screening; what you get will depend on your country, where you live, and your health insurance plan, where applicable.

Genetic screening of the fetus has advanced dramatically over the last three decades, and continues to change almost yearly. Keeping up with the latest set of tests and standards can be a challenge. Many women are surprised how quickly things are changing, even from their first pregnancy to the next.

This chapter will explain the basic concepts behind the testing you are likely to be offered. There may be some subtle differences from region to region and country to country, but after reading this chapter you will have a general understanding of the current screening methods that you are likely to encounter.

What is high risk?

A pregnancy is considered at high risk if the odds of having a chromosomally abnormal baby are found to be higher than 1 in approximately 250.

Genetic *screening* is the method by which your care provider attempts to find those pregnancies that are at a higher risk for being chromosomally abnormal. If you are found to be at higher risk, it does not mean your baby IS abnormal, but it does mean you may wish to consider genetic testing. Genetic screening poses absolutely no risk to the fetus. In contrast to screening, genetic *testing* is the only definitive way to be sure that your fetus has the proper number of chromosomes. Genetic testing requires that a sample of fetal tissue be obtained and analyzed. Obtaining fetal tissue is performed via an amniocentesis or a chorionic villus sampling (CVS) and poses a small but real risk of causing a miscarriage, which is fully explained in the next chapter.

The balancing act of screening

A good screening test will find as many abnormal pregnancies as possible, while at the same time avoiding erroneously labelling normal pregnancies as high risk. Flagging a normal pregnancy as being at high risk is called a *false positive*, while missing an abnormal pregnancy is known as a *false negative*. A good way to appreciate the complexity of this challenge is to picture a large jar of marbles. The majority of the marbles are white (normal pregnancies) but there are some red marbles (abnormal pregnancies) scattered randomly throughout. There is only a barely discernable difference between the white and red marbles, and we need to design a task that is going to capture as many of those red marbles as possible. If we scoop out a large portion of the jar, we will probably catch quite a few of the red marbles, maybe only leaving a couple behind, but we will also grab a lot of white marbles unnecessarily. Alternatively, if we wish to reduce the number of white marbles we pick up, we could take a smaller sample size, but we will probably miss most of the reds. Ideally, we need to devise a way to catch ONLY the red marbles and discard all of the whites. This is the challenge in desiging a good screening test: to increase the detection rate of abnormal fetuses to as close to 100% as possible, while at the same time maintaining a low false positive rate.

Maternal age

In the 1970s and the 1980s, it was well understood that the likelihood of having a baby with Down's syndrome increased with age. Maternal age therefore became the sole basis on which health care providers would offer genetic testing. In general, the line between low and high risk was drawn at 35–37 years old. However, because Down's syndrome babies can be born to a woman of ANY age, and because the majority of women having babies are under 35 years old, the majority of babies born with Down's syndrome are born to women under 35. Offering amniocentesis (amnio) to each woman over 35 meant that some abnormal babies were found, but the majority of Down's syndrome babies were still being missed. Furthermore, using age 35–37 as the sole filtering criterion meant that the vast majority of amnios were done on perfectly normal babies. Going back to the jar analogy, using age alone catches a lot of white marbles to find only a small portion of the reds. It became clear that using age alone is not an ideal method of screening.

Serum screening

In the 1990s, links were detected between altered concentrations of some pregnancy-related chemicals in the blood and abnormal chromosomes. The relative amounts of these chemicals could also indicate which type of chromosomal abnormality might be present. This was very exciting: now every woman, regardless of her age, can more accurately discover her risk status. It is currently possible to detect prenatally the majority of Down's syndrome and other chromosomally abnormal cases in all age groups. The three most common type of chromosomal abnormalities are trisomy 21 (also known as Down's syndrome), trisomy 13, and trisomy 18. Trisomy 13 and 18 are almost always lethal, and 80% of fetuses affected will die in the womb between 12 and 40 weeks. Those that do survive to term usually die shortly after birth. Trisomy 21 (Down's syndrome) is not lethal, and although there can be some severe anatomical defects associated with it, most Down's syndrome babies that do not miscarry can be expected to survive well until adulthood.

Initially, screening for these trisomies was done by looking for markers in a sample of the mother's blood taken at approximately 16 weeks gestation. Eventually, the 'triple' and 'quad' screen tests emerged as the standard, and are still used today. These blood tests will appropriately flag 55–80% of fetuses with trisomy 21, but they have a false positive rate of at least 5% (some studies

What is tested in the quad screen?

- **AFP (alpha fetoprotein):** produced by the fetus, elevated levels can also indicate an open spinal or abdominal defect

- **hCG (human chorionic gonadotropin:** produced by the placenta

- **Estriol:** an estrogen, produced by fetus and placenta

- **Inhibin-A:** a protein, produced by placenta and maternal ovaries.

The triple screen

Tests for all of the above, minus the Inhibin A.

indicate a false positive rate for the triple/quad screen as high as 10%.) This does not mean that 5% of those that get a positive result have an abnormal baby, but rather that 5% of ALL women who receive the test will be told they are high risk and yet are really carrying a perfectly normal baby. In contrast, the true incidence of Down's syndrome is only about 0.25% or quarter of 1%. We want to stress this because it means that if you are found to be at high risk, do not panic. The chances are still very good that your baby is normal.

The triple and quad screen has been replaced by combined nuchal translucency (NT) and first trimester testing (explained in the next section) in many localities, but is still used if the mother misses the window for earlier testing. This sometimes happens in cases where a woman didn't realize she was pregnant before 14 weeks, or where there was a lack of access to earlier prenatal care. Whether the triple screen or the quad screen is used depends upon the area where you live and your maternity care scheme. The quad screen is a slightly more accurate test than the triple screen, but the difference is minimal. A penta screen is currently being developed and used in select areas to further improve accuracy, with the hopes of eventually replacing the triple/quad.

First trimester integrated testing

Continued research into improving the detection rate of fetal abnormalities has led to the development of multi-factorial screening. This means that multiple factors are combined to assess risk (hence the term 'integrated'). First trimester integrated screening combines the evaluation of chemical markers in the maternal blood with maternal age, ultrasound measurements of the nuchal translucency, and fetal age. There are different names for this test (First Screen,

UltraScreen, etc) depending on where you have the test, but they are all variations of the same technique. A full explanation of what happens at the ultrasound scan portion of the test is described in Chapter 8; in brief, a measurement is taken of a thin pocket of fluid located just under the skin behind the fetal neck, called the nuchal translucency or NT. During the ultrasound scan, the length of the baby from head to rump is also measured in order to establish an accurate gestational age. In some places providers will also take measurements of the fetal nasal bone and heart rate. The chemical markers in the mother's blood that are examined in the screening are beta-hCG, which is produced by the placenta, and pregnancy-associated plasma protein A (PAPP-A). All these factors are combined using sophisticated multivariate statistical techniques to arrive at a general, combined risk ratio.

First trimester integrated testing has been widely adopted, since it has a better detection rate than the triple or quad screen, (approx 88–95% accurate) and a lower false positive rate. Best of all, the results are obtained by the end of the first trimester when detection and possible intervention is preferable.

Variations on the first trimester integrated screening

- **Sequential screen:** This type of testing involves doing an integrated first trimester screen at 12 weeks and following it up with a triple or quad screen (or penta) at 16 weeks. A preliminary report is generated after the first screen, with a final report given after the second screen is processed.

- **Contingency screening:** An integrated first trimester screen is done at 12 weeks. If the result is found to be at moderate or intermediate risk where the ratio is between 1 in 50 to 1 in 2000, then a triple, quad, or penta sample will be drawn to get a final result.

- **How accurate are these tests?** Depending on the lab and the supporting data, variations of the First Trimester Integrated Screen generally yield an approximately 88–95% detection rate with a false positive rate of 2–5%.

All the possible variations of the possible screening tests available make it hard to predict exactly which protocol you will receive. The reason there are so many possibilities is that there are multiple groups of researchers and laboratories: each are trying to come up with the most accurate test, which will detect the highest percentage of abnormal fetuses, with the lowest false positive rate. Independent studies of each lab's test often yield slightly different results, meaning that there are likely to be some inconsistencies in numbers quoted for screening test accuracy rates. The accuracy statistics you are given may be slightly different from what is presented here.

In countries where there is a single entity that establishes national health standards, the type of screening protocol available to the population is likely to be based on a predetermined national guideline. Other women may have a health care scheme or insurance plan that specifies which type(s) of testing is(are) reimbursable. Ultimately, you may not be offered a choice as to which type of screening you would prefer to receive, but the differences in accuracy between the various methods are very small.

FAQ: 'How long do I have to wait for my results?' If you have a triple, quad, or penta screen, your blood will be drawn at 16 weeks and results can take up to one week. If you have integrated first trimester screening, your blood can be drawn at any point from 10–13 weeks, and the ultrasound needs to be done between 11 and 13.6 weeks. Some places will draw the blood at the same time as the ultrasound, or they may do the blood test a week or two earlier. Either way, the results will be available usually within the same day to a week after the ultrasound is performed. If you have the sequential screening, where an additional blood draw is taken at 16 weeks, then your final result will be available within the week after that.

What the integrated results look like

The lab will generate a report that is sent to your provider, which will break down your risks based on the various factors and give a total, cumulative risk ratio. A typical report contains the following information.

Patient name: xxxxxxxxxxxx

Age at EDD: 26

CRL–56.2 mm. = 12W1D

Risk table	Down's syndrome	Trisomy 18/13
1 Maternal Age (26)	1 in 912	1 in 1 616
2 Age + Biochemistry	1 in 905	1 in >10 000
3 Nuchal Translucency	1 in 4 914	1 in >10 000
4 Age + Biochem + NT	**1 in 4 877**	**1 in >10 000**
Results	**Within range**	**Within range**

Age at EDD (estimated date of delivery/birth or estimated due date) means the age that the mother will be when she is due to deliver the baby. CRL stands for 'crown rump length' and determines the age of the fetus, in this case corresponding to 12 weeks and 1 day. Line 1 shows that the general, background risk of any 26 year old having a baby with Down's syndrome is 1 in 912 and the risk of a trisomy 18 or 13 baby is 1 in 1616. On line 2, the risk is recalculated using age plus the biochemistry (blood test results), which shows that the risk didn't increase or decrease significantly for Down's Syndrome, but the risk for trisomy 18 or 13 improved dramatically to less than 1 in 10,000 (which is the upper limit of the odds that are possible). Line 3 shows the patient's risk based solely on the NT thickness (which was 0.9 mm), which is a very reassuring 1 in 4914 for Down's syndrome and again, an excellent result for trisomy 18/13. Finally, line 4 is the integrated, cumulative risk value combining the age, biochemistry, and NT measurement. The overall risk that this woman is carrying a fetus with Down's syndrome is 1 in 4,877 and there is a less than 1 in 10,000 risk of her having a Trisomy 13/18 fetus. This woman is well below the 1 in 250 cutoff for higher risk status.

The next case demonstrates how screening tests can adjust the risk ratio of an 'advanced age' woman, to help them decide whether or not they want to pursue invasive testing.

Patient name: xxxxxxxxxxxxx

Age at EDD: 39

CRL–60.1 mm. = 12W2D

Risk table	Down's syndrome	Trisomy 18/13
1 Maternal Age (39)	1 in 93	1 in 166
2 Age + Biochemistry	1 in 658	1 in >6 230
3 Nuchal Translucency	1 in 1 348	1 in >1 155
4 Age + Biochem + NT	**1 in 1 841**	**1 in >3 301**
Results	**Within range**	**Within range**

Based on her age of 39, this woman has a general background risk of having a Down's syndrome baby of 1 in 93, and a 1 in 166 chance of trisomy 18/13. However, when all the testing factors are combined, her overall Down's risk is revised to 1 in 1841, which is similar to the general risk of a 21 year old. These are very reassuring results, but they serve as a reminder that relying on screening is comparable to gambling. It's a game of playing the odds and hoping that you are not that 1 out of 1,841. In addition, there are a small number of people who have an abnormal fetus that will slip through the screening (known as false negatives). Because older women do have a higher risk of abnormal fetuses, rather than gambling that they are not going to be one of those few that are missed, they still have the option to pursue invasive testing, to be assured of 100% accuracy in detection.

What a positive result looks like

Patient name: xxxxxxxxxxxxx

Age at EDD: 31

CRL–64.7 mm. = 12W5D

Risk table	Down's syndrome	Trisomy 18/13
1 Maternal Age (31)	1 in 555	1 in 974
2 Age + Biochemistry	1 in 29	1 in >10 000
3 Nuchal Translucency	1 in 2 521	1 in >7 874
4 Age + Biochem + NT	**1 in 130**	**1 in >10 000**
Results	****Increased risk****	**Within range**

Based solely on the woman's age of 31, she is at a low background risk to be carrying an abnormal fetus. However, when the results of the blood test are factored in, her risk that the fetus could be affected with Down's syndrome significantly increases to 1 in 29. Her fetal nuchal translucency result of 1.6 mm (not shown) is reassuring when taken in isolation, giving an overall Down's risk of 1 in 2521. However, when all the factors are combined, the overall results show that this woman has an **overall risk ratio of 1 in 130**. This demonstrates that the parameters are weighted differently, with the serum results increasing the overall risk despite a reassuring age and a normal NT. This result puts this woman in the 'increased risk' category for Down's syndrome, because 1 in 130 is higher than the cutoff of 1 in 250. It makes sense for this 31 year old to consider further testing with CVS or amniocentesis.

FAQ: 'My screening test is positive and I am being sent to a specialist to have a level II ultrasound. Will they be able to tell me if my baby is OK?' A complete, targeted anatomy scan is also known as a level II ultrasound and is often performed by a perinatologist, who is a maternal fetal medicine specialist. These specialists are well trained to handle higher risk and complicated pregnancies. Should your screening test be positive, you may be sent to a specialty centre where a complete evaluation of the fetal anatomy will be performed. If the fetus is shown to have any anatomical abnormalities, this will increase the suspicion that the baby might suffer from a chromosomal abnormality. Depending on the abnormality (or abnormalities) found, the doctor will be able to revise your risk ratio and discuss your options with you. You will almost certainly be offered an amniocentesis or CVS, depending on the gestational age of the pregnancy.

It is likely that the ultrasound scan will find that the fetus looks perfectly normal. While this is reassuring, there is absolutely no way to be certain that this fetus does not have a problem without performing an invasive genetic test. An important fact: many Down's syndrome babies will appear completely normal on ultrasound. If your screening test is positive and you have a normal ultrasound, you are still a candidate for an amniocentesis or CVS.

FAQ: 'A while back, my sister's screening test showed her at high risk, but she gave birth to a beautiful healthy baby. It was so frightening for all of us. After all that unnecessary anxiety, I'm wondering if I should even do the screening?' Early versions of screening tests had an unfortunately high rate of false positives, meaning that woman found to be high risk on the screening test would often still have a normal baby. Many women got the upsetting test result that they might be carrying a baby with a problem, and many thousands of amniocentesis proceduress were done on perfectly healthy pregnancies. As the screening tests have improved, the false-positive rates have fallen. Fewer women are getting that frightening news than ever before, but unfortunately, the perfect screening test doesn't exist yet. Despite using the latest screening techniques, these scares still happen every day.

You always have the option to refuse the screening, which makes perfect sense if you would not consider doing an invasive test like amniocentesis, or terminating the pregnancy, even if the baby is abnormal. Refusing the screening will spare you the next 6 months of waiting and worrying until the baby is born to discover if the positive screening result was legitimate. However, if you want to know for any reason if you are indeed at higher risk, then you should probably consent to being screened. Rather than being consumed with worry and anxiety, remember that the majority of babies that are flagged as high risk during screening turn out to be perfectly healthy and normal.

The future of screening and testing

The information presented in this chapter and the next are likely to become obsolete within the not-too-distant future, perhaps within this coming decade. New technologies are being developed that will allow for non-invasive diagnostic testing using circulating cell-free DNA that can be collected from the mother's blood. With a simple blood sample taken from the mother, it will become possible to do DNA analysis of the fetus and rule out Down's syndrome, other chromosomal abnormalities, and many other genetic diseases. Obtaining this information from a maternal blood sample means that a fetal diagnosis could be obtained without the risk of harming the pregnancy with an invasive test. The technology itself is not too far from being a reality; however, it will be a while before it becomes available to the general population. It will be very expensive, especially initially, so assessment of risk versus cost will need to be considered. There will many other details that will need to be addressed, including the ethical implications of being able to obtain detailed information early on in the development of the fetus. For instance, in addition to assessing the chromosomes, this information will include fetal sex, and disease carrier status. One thing that is certain is that there will continue to be exciting and dramatic developments in fetal screening and testing in the future.

4

Genetic testing of the fetus

➲ Key points

◆ Genetic testing obtains fetal chromosomes for analysis, giving a definitive diagnosis of normal versus abnormal chromosomes.

◆ Medical indications for genetic testing include advanced maternal age, positive results on screening tests, or anatomical abnormalities found on ultrasound.

◆ Unlike screening, genetic testing is an invasive procedure that carries a small risk of causing a miscarriage.

◆ The two most common methods for genetic testing are amniocentesis and chorionic villus sampling (CVS).

◆ General chromosomal analysis gives detail only on the structure and number of chromosomes of the fetus. Additional specialized testing can be performed in patients who are found to be at a very high risk for specific disorders.

In order to definitively identify whether or not your baby has a chromosomal abnormality, a sample of the fetus's genetic material must be obtained. The only way this can currently be done is to physically extract a tissue sample from the fetus, either by amniocentesis (putting a needle into the amniotic sac to draw out amniotic fluid) or chorionic villus sampling (putting a needle into the developing placenta to draw out a sample of tissue). Both tests have the potential to introduce infection, or cause rupture of membranes or premature labour leading to loss of the pregnancy. Couples need to make an informed decision about whether taking this small risk is personally acceptable to them.

Why might you be offered invasive testing?

When considering whether or not invasive testing is appropriate, your provider weighs the risks of an amniocentesis or CVS against the odds that your baby has a problem. In other words, is the likelihood that there is a genetic abnormality with the fetus great enough to consider putting the pregnancy at risk by doing this procedure? Until recently, women were advised that the risk of losing the pregnancy following amniocentesis was approximately 0.5%. In the United Kingdom, the accepted risk quoted is 1 in 200, while in the U.S. the standard quote is 1 in 300. To simplify, we will use 1 in 250 in this discussion. These numbers are based on data from studies done back in the 1970's, before it was routine to use ultrasound guidance during amniocentesis, and before doctors had amassed expertise with the procedure. Over the last two decades, clinical experience suggests that the 1 in 200 risk has been greatly overestimated, since actual pregnancy loss following a procedure is rare. However, it is still standard practice to refer to these older statistics and to use the oft-quoted number of approximately 1 in 250. The risks associated with CVS are thought to be about 1 in 100.

What is it about being 35 years old or older that suddenly prompts your provider to suggest that you opt for amniocentesis or CVS, even if you've had prior normal pregnancies? Nothing dramatic happens to a woman's eggs on her 35th birthday compared to her 34th. However, the general statistical risk of having a baby with a genetic abnormality at age 35 now rises to more than 1 in 300, specifically 1 in approximately 278. It is at this point of turning 35 years old that the risk of having a baby with a chromosomal problem becomes higher than the risk of having a miscarriage from undergoing an amniocentesis (according to U.S. standards). In the United Kingdom, because the medically established risk quoted for an amniocentesis is 1 in 200, it is considered appropriate to offer invasive testing once a woman is older than 37, as the odds of having a baby with Down's syndrome are then approximately 1 in 180.

With the advent of serum screening tests (described in Chapter 3) and targeted early ultrasounds (described in Chapter 7), it became possible to identify fetuses at a higher risk for Down's syndrome, trisomy 13 and 18, and other chromosomal abnormalities, regardless of the mother's age. This screening is offered to ALL pregnant women of all ages since the vast majority (80%) of Down's syndrome babies are born to women under 35. The screening tests are considered positive if the total risk is calculated to be greater than 1 in approximately 250, i.e. similar to or higher than the risk of an invasive procedure. However, we cannot stress enough that even if the screening test is positive, it does not mean the fetus has a chromosomal problem. Most women who are flagged as high risk are carrying a perfectly normal child. However, your provider will offer you further testing as it is now deemed medically appropriate.

Medical indications for amniocentesis or cvs

◈ Advanced maternal age (>35 in the US, >37 in the UK)

◈ Family history of specific genetic disorders

◈ Prior pregnancy with specific disorders

◈ Screening results are 'positive', indicating a greater than 1 in 250 chance that a genetic abnormality may be present

As mentioned above, the 1 in 250 (0.4%) estimate for the risk of pregnancy loss with an invasive procedure is not a definitive figure. In 2006, a database of over 35,000 women who participated in the Mt. Sinai School of Medicine FASTER Trial (First And Second Trimester Evaluation of Risk for Aneuploidy) was analyzed. Based on these data, researchers concluded that the risk of pregnancy loss from amniocentesis was around 1 in 1600 (0.06%). However, other contemporary studies could not replicate the FASTER trial's impressive results, and most researchers are doubtful that the risk is really that low. Most current studies conclude that the real rate most likely lies somewhere between 1 in 1200 and 1 in 300 (0.08% and 0.33%). The exact rate of miscarriage is still being debated, but the overall message is that the risk is likely to be lower than that traditionally quoted. These results show that using risk of miscarriage alone as the benchmark for offering invasive testing may not be optimal. That is, it may not be ideal to balance the risk of having an abnormal baby on the one hand, versus the risk of a miscarriage from testing on the other. Modern medicine is in the process of assimilating all this new data into practice, and this makes for uncertainty regarding when invasive testing is truly appropriate. If we were to use the most optimistic miscarriage risk of 1 in 1600 as the criterion to determine who should be offered an amniocentesis, then we'd have to offer it to almost everyone as the general risk of a Down's syndrome baby for a 21-year-old is approximately 1 in 1520 pregnancies. Does it make any sense to offer an amniocentesis to anyone over 21, just because she's slightly more likely to have a baby with Down's syndrome than she is to have a miscarriage from an amniocentesis? Certainly not, as even a loss rate as small as 0.06% is significant. Consider these numbers: in 2008, there were just under 5,000,000 babies born in the UK and the US combined. If an amniocentesis was done in every pregnancy, a loss rate of 0.06% translates to 3,000 miscarriages in that one year, the overwhelming majority of which would have been normal babies. A loss rate of 1 in 250 or 0.4% would mean 200,000 miscarriages.

Balancing the Risks

To decide whether or not invasive testing is indicated, the risk of causing a miscarriage by inserting a needle is balanced against the likelihood of the baby having a chromosomal problem.

Doctors cannot offer invasive testing to everyone as it is too risky and costly. It still makes good common sense to use that 1 in 250 point as the cutoff for low risk versus increased risk. Statistics and numbers aside, the important thing is to understand exactly how this all applies to you as a patient, your partner, and your unborn baby. Data shows that in recent years, the number of people opting to undergo invasive testing procedures has dropped thanks to the increased confidence in the NT and first and second trimester blood work. However, not all older women are comfortable relying on the screening tests, and with good reason. At present, false negatives on screening occur 6 to 10% of the time. A false negative occurs when the screening test is normal, but the baby is in fact abnormal. In other words, present screening tests will flag 90 to 94 abnormal babies out of every 100 chromosomally abnormal babies. Those are pretty good odds, and many people are comfortable with that level of assurance. However, it also means that 6 to 10 chromosomally abnormal babies will be missed by the screening, and many people feel that is too many. If you want to know with 100% certainty that your baby does not have Down's syndrome or another chromosomal abnormality, the only way to get a definitive answer is to opt for an invasive diagnostic test, i.e. amnio or CVS. This is a very personal decision with no right or wrong answer. Your provider's role is to tell you if you are in a higher risk category and to let you know if you are medically eligible for further testing. Many people interpret this as being told that their provider wants them to have the test, but he or she is only doing their job by letting you know your risks and options. It is your choice whether or not you want to proceed with further testing.

CVS versus amniocentesis

Chorionic villus sampling (CVS) is performed at the end of the first trimester, between 10.5 and 13 weeks, and amniocentesis can be performed at any point after 16 weeks. While getting results earlier in the pregnancy is very appealing, CVS has not replaced amniocentesis as the most prevalent method of testing because the risk of a loss may be slightly higher. In addition, expertise in the technique is limited to high-risk specialty practices, which makes access to

CVS more challenging in many locations. There are simply fewer doctors trained and experienced enough to do them. The loss-risk for CVS is traditionally quoted as being approximately 1%, or 1 in 100. Again, current practice suggests that the actual number of losses is lower than that, especially in expert hands, but no recent study data are available to revise the figure officially. A study done in 2006 at the University of California, San Francisco compared 20 years of amniocentesis and CVS data. The researchers found that, over the *entire* period, average loss rates between the two tests were roughly the same, but there was a noticeable decrease over 15 years in the loss rate from CVS. This reflects the medical learning curve, as CVS was a relatively new test, and proficiency in performing this intervention is critical to a successful outcome. There have also been reports of an additional (albeit small) correlation of CVS with the occurrence of limb defects in the developing fetus, for reasons that are not fully understood. In reviewing those findings, it was felt that the timing of CVS was a factor (with the risk being increased if the test was performed at less than 10.5 weeks). As a result, CVS is no longer performed routinely before 10.5 weeks, and the associated incidence of limb defects is now quite rare.

Advantage of CVS:

- It is performed between 10.5 and 13 weeks, allowing for earlier diagnosis

Advantage of amniocentesis:

- Large window of time, as it can be done any time after 16 weeks

- Fluid can be tested for elevated alpha-fetoprotein (AFP), which can signal the presence of a spinal or abdominal defect. However, these defects would usually be detected by ultrasound.

The ability to obtain a genetic diagnosis with CVS at the end of the first trimester has a distinct advantage over a 16-week amniocentesis. It is preferable to know sooner rather than later if the fetus does have a chromosomal problem. If a problem is found, the woman has the option of an earlier termination (abortion), which has lower complication rates and can be less emotionally traumatic than terminating a pregnancy later on. In addition, knowing that there is a problem before the pregnancy is 'showing' allows for greater privacy.

Amniocentesis has an advantage over CVS in that they both check the chromosomes, but the amniotic fluid can also be tested for the level of AFP (alpha-fetoprotein). Abnormal levels of AFP in the amniotic fluid can indicate an open spinal or brain defect such as spina bifida, or an abnormal opening in the abdomen, known as gastroschisis. In these cases, the fetus may be genetically normal but still suffer from a severe anatomical defect. However, this advantage of amniocentesis over CVS has lessened, owing to advances in ultrasound imaging. Most of these defects can and will be discovered during routine ultrasound screening between 16 and 20 weeks gestation.

What to expect if you are having an amniocentesis or CVS

If a woman is of advanced maternal age (a politically correct yet unpopular term for pregnant women who are age 35/37 or older), has a family history of genetic abnormality, or is flagged during routine blood and NT screening, then genetic counselling and fetal chromosomal studies will be offered. Ultrasound plays an integral role in guiding physicians to obtain samples of genetic material for chromosomal analysis. The two methods available with current technologies are chorionic villus sampling (CVS) and amniocentesis. The indications and associated risks of the two procedures are described above. This section discusses the practical aspects of each test.

Amniocentesis

The amniocentesis procedure is performed around 16 weeks gestation, and while it may sound scary and painful, it is relatively simple and usually only mildly uncomfortable. An amniocentesis is performed in order to remove a sample of the amniotic fluid which surrounds the fetus. Amniotic fluid is normally a light yellow-coloured liquid that the fetus swallows, processes through the intestines, kidneys, and bladder, and then eliminates. It is essentially 'urine', but since most of the waste products of the fetus pass through the umbilical cord and through the mother, it can be regarded as a sterile recycled fluid. Floating in the fluid are cells from the fetal skin, intestinal tract, and bladder, which the fetus has sloughed off. The lab is able to harvest these cells from the fluid and grow them (called tissue culture) to yield the chromosomes that will be analyzed.

Amniocentesis is done using ultrasound guidance. Before the procedure begins, you will be scanned abdominally and some measurements of the fetus will probably be performed. The uterus will be assessed for an easily accessible pocket of amniotic fluid. The doctor and sonographer or assistant will be working together, and once they are confident that an open path into the fluid is available, preparation begins. Preparation takes much longer than the procedure itself. Your abdomen will be cleaned with an antiseptic solution, and the doctor will set up a sterile field and put on sterile gloves. A sterile shield is placed over the ultrasound probe and sterile gel is applied. Anaesthetic (novacaine/lidocaine) was commonly used in the past, but many facilities no longer bother. Arguably, the anaesthetic is actually more painful than the amniocentesis itself, because it requires an additional needle stick and the lidocaine tends to burn before it takes effect. Additionally, if the doctor takes the time to anaesthetize the area, there is a chance that the baby might move and the spot might no longer be open, so the whole numbing process would have to start again somewhere else. The decision whether to give a local anaesthetic is usually based on the personal preferences of the doctor performing the test. Rest assured that whether or not you get anaesthetic, it is not going to make much of difference to the minimal discomfort you are likely to experience.

Once everything is sterile and ready, another look is taken with the ultrasound probe. If the fetus is still cooperating and hasn't moved into the pocket of fluid, the doctor will insert the needle while watching the live image on the ultrasound monitor. Some doctors prefer to use a needle guide attached to the probe to help direct the needle, others prefer to work free-hand. If the baby gets in the way, or the pocket no longer looks optimal, the doctor can stop, look around, and pick a better approach. Getting the needle into the pocket usually happens very quickly, and the woman often only feels a strange

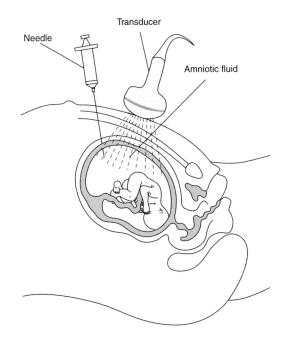

pressure sensation. Once the needle is in the fluid, the doctor slides the stylet (the centre of the needle) out, leaving a very thin, hollow tube. At this point, even if the fetus comes into contact with the needle, it's not going to be injured and will usually move away reflexively. A syringe is attached to the base of the needle and fluid is drawn out, about 20 mL or 4 teaspoons is typical. The fetus isn't affected by the loss of fluid, as the amount taken is usually less than 10% of the overall fluid volume and is quickly replaced by the fetus and placenta. A very thin needle is used to minimize injury to the uterus and amniotic sac, so it can take up to a minute to draw enough fluid through the narrow opening. Women usually feel very little discomfort while the fluid is being drawn, perhaps some pressure. The needle is then removed, and the fluid is transferred to tubes and sent to the lab where it will be analyzed. Most patients find that waiting 10 to 14 days for the results is much harder than the procedure itself.

CVS

Instead of sampling amniotic fluid, chorionic villus sampling or CVS involves the retrieval of cells from early placental tissue known as chorionic villi. The main advantage of CVS versus amniocentesis is that it is performed between 10.5 and 13 weeks, and therefore can give an earlier diagnosis. Like an amniocentesis, the procedure will be performed in a sterile environment under ultrasound guidance, but it can be done in one of two ways: through the abdomen, or transvaginally through the cervix, known as trans-cervical CVS. You will be instructed to arrive for your appointment with a full bladder, which is usually essential if the procedure is to be done vaginally. Your doctor will make the decision as to which approach to take, based on the location of the placenta and the position of your uterus. You will not have much of a choice about abdominal versus vaginal CVS, as this decision is best left to the doctor's experience and preference. If the doctor chooses a cervical approach, you will need to be undressed from the waist down, lie on your back, with your legs apart. A speculum will be inserted into the vaginal canal so that the doctor can get a good view of the cervix. Usually, the pressure of the speculum on a full bladder is the most uncomfortable thing about this procedure. An antiseptic solution will be liberally applied, which is painless. Sometimes the doctor will use an instrument to grab hold of the cervix, in which case you will feel a pinch. A soft flexible catheter is inserted with a bendable metal stylet through the cervical canal. A sonographer will be simultaneously scanning the abdomen with the ultrasound probe, allowing the doctor to direct the path of the catheter towards the optimum spot. Once the catheter is in the desired location, the doctor slides it back and forth a few times to collect the tissue. The catheter is then withdrawn, the retrieved cells will be squirted into a vial, and the sample will be checked under a microscope to ensure that enough tissue was obtained. Sometimes, a second or third pass may be required in order to obtain enough cells for the lab to successfully culture.

Rather than going transcervically, the doctor may want to take a trans abdominal approach, depending on where the placenta is growing. In this case, the procedure is very similar to an amniocentesis, except that instead of collecting amniotic fluid, samples of the placental tissue will be taken. Whether CVS is done abdominally or vaginally, the procedure is usually very well tolerated, causing very little pain. Most women find the full bladder to be the worst part of the experience.

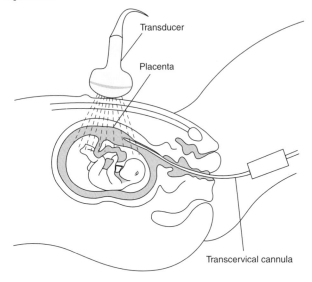

Transducer

Placenta

Transcervical cannula

Things to expect after an amniocentesis or CVS

Following either procedure, your doctor will likely instruct you to take it easy for at least 24 hours, avoiding strenuous physical activity and sexual intercourse. Strict bed rest is unnecessary, but this is not the day to run loads of laundry up and down the stairs or carry your toddler through the shops. Try to have a relaxing day. Call your provider if you experience any vaginal bleeding, severe cramping, a temperature of 38.0°C (100.4°F) or greater, or leakage of fluid from the vagina. If you had an amniocentesis or abdominal CVS, the fluid will never leak from the spot where the needle went into the abdomen, as that hole closes immediately. If you had a transcervical CVS, spotting and even some red bleeding for a few days afterwards is to be <u>expected</u>. Sexual intercourse and tampon use should be avoided until this resolves. It is always frightening for women to see any bleeding during pregnancy, but this is normal following a transcervical CVS, so try not to panic. Call your provider if the bleeding becomes heavy or is associated with painful cramps. Other symptoms to watch for include fever, vaginal leakage of amniotic fluid, or severe cramping without bleeding. Call your provider if any of those things occur or if you have any other concerns. Most of the time, even if you do experience some of these complications, things will resolve within a few days and the pregnancy continues forward without further problems.

Many patients assume that if something were to go wrong, it would happen during the procedure itself, but this is almost never the case. If a miscarriage were to occur, symptoms would become evident within the first 48 hours after the CVS or amniocentesis. Anything that happens within two weeks after any procedure would be considered procedure-related. However, spontaneous losses can and do occur at any point in a pregnancy, even without invasive testing, and it is almost impossible to tell whether you would have miscarried anyway.

Can an amniocentesis or CVS be done on twins?

Both procedures can be done on twins, triplets, or even more. With amniocentesis, the doctor may choose to inject a small amount of harmless blue dye back into the sac of the first fetus after the sample is taken. The entire procedure is then repeated for the second or subsequent sacs. When a fresh sample of fluid is drawn, it should be the normal light-yellow color and not blue-tinged. This ensures that each gestation is sampled separately. With three or more fetuses, obtaining tissue from each becomes more difficult and is not always possible for every fetus, depending on their locations within the uterus. Research data suggest that the miscarriage rates for amniocentesis or CVS go up when the procedures are performed on twins or multiple pregnancies. Testing on multiple pregnancies will probably be done at a high-risk centre by high-risk obstetricians (perinatologists), who will be able to discuss your risks and options with you based on your individual situation, and the number and location of gestations.

If you are rhesus negative (Rh−)

Your doctor should know your blood type before doing any interventional procedures. If you are Rh−, you will require an injection of anti-D or Rhogam, which will prevent your body from developing antibodies against any fetal blood cells that may enter your system. These antibodies produced by the mother can cross the placenta and attack the red blood cells of the fetus if the fetus is Rh+. This can lead to a syndrome of severe fetal anaemia, a scenario which is fortunately avoidable with a prophylactic dose of anti-D/Rhogam.

Analysis and the results

CVS and amniocentesis both allow for the fetal chromosomes to be isolated and analyzed, a process known as cytogenetics or karyotyping. When sperm and egg combine, each should contribute 23 chromosomes so that an embryo with 46 chromosomes begins to grow. All humans should have 23 pairs of chromosomes, half contributed by the mother and the other half from the father. The 23rd set determines the sex of the fetus, with an XX being female and XY being male. Cytogenetic results will always identify the sex of the fetus, but you can choose whether or not you want to be told. In order to study the chromosomes, the lab isolates the fetal cells from the specimen (be it amniotic fluid or chorionic villi) and places them in an incubator to culture them. The cells have to be properly cultured to a point where they are ready to divide, as it is only at this point that chromosomes are visible within the cell nucleus. Once they are isolated, the chromosomes are dyed so they can be better visualized, examined, and photographed under a microscope. Because the cell culture that has to grow, the process cannot be hurried, and the timing of the results can vary. Usually the process is complete within 7 to 10 days, and a final report is generated within 2 weeks.

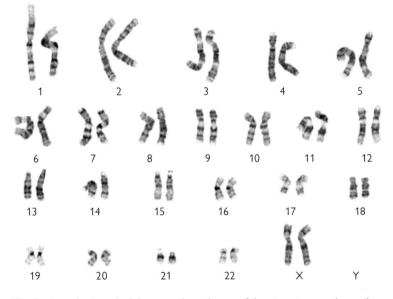

The final result gives the lab a complete picture of the **structure** and **number** of the fetal chromosomes. Some specific inherited diseases like cystic fibrosis or Tay-Sachs can be detected but this type of targeted testing is only performed if there is a known high risk. Any disorder that results from having too many or too few chromosomes will be detected. This includes (but is not limited to) Down's syndrome, also known as trisomy 21, where an extra chromosome is present at the 21st pair. In addition, the overall structure of the chromosomes is reviewed, to detect whether any portion of a chromosome is missing or broken. It is important to understand that general cytogenetic studies do not detect every type of genetic disease, they only look at the structure and number of the chromosomes of your fetus. Any disorder that involves too many, too few, incomplete, or rearranged chromosomes will be revealed, but it does not expose what lies *within* the thousands of genes that comprise the chromosomes. There are about 25,000 to 35,000 genes within the 46 chromosomes, half of which are contributed by the mother and the other half by the father. The myriad of gene combinations determine the individual traits a person has such as eye colour, height, blood type and so on. Within these genes can also lie certain inherited genetic diseases such as hoemophilia, cystic fibrosis, and diabetes to name just a few. In a routine amniocentesis or CVS, only the structure and number of chromosomes are studied and they will <u>not</u> show inherited diseases hiding within the genes. This means that a normal amniocentesis does not guarantee a perfectly healthy child.

What if my results are abnormal?

If the testing reveals that your baby has an abnormal number of chromosomes, or a chromosome structural defect, you will be offered genetic counselling. Too many or too few chromosomes usually results in physical birth defects and mental retardation. Abnormalities within the structure or rearrangement of chromosomes can cause problems of varying degree, ranging from minimal to severe. In the case of rearrangements, genetic material may be seen to be evenly swapped between 2 chromosomes, not affecting the overall gene coding. This is known as a balanced translocation. Usually, this has no significance on the child's development or intelligence. In fact, further testing of the parents will very often show that one of them possesses the exact same translocation. Unbalanced translocations occur when the swapping of genetic material between chromosomes is unequal, resulting in extra or missing genes. In these cases, fetal development is almost always affected negatively, and serious abnormalities and intellectual impairments are probable. There are a number of anomalies associated with the sex chromosomes, which can have subtle to severe effects. Some sex chromosome abnormalities can allow normal development of the child, but cause infertility in adulthood. No matter what the test reveals, most of the irregularities that can occur are well studied. Should you have an abnormal result of any kind, you will be referred to a geneticist or genetic counsellor who will be able to provide you with information regarding the prognosis, probabilities, and types of impairments associated with that specific disorder. You will also be advised as to your options for termination, or for special care that might be required before, during and after birth if you choose to continue the pregnancy.

I was told I'm a carrier for cystic fibrosis. Will the results show if my baby has the disease?

Generally, an amniocentesis or CVS doesn't look for cystic fibrosis or any other problem other than the structure and number of chromosomes. If there a strong family history for a known inherited disease, or if the prenatal screening uncovers that both parents are carriers of a disease (see Chapter III, *Genetic Screening of the Parents*), it is possible for the lab to look for the corresponding mutation within the fetal chromosomes. Some of the diseases that can be detected with today's technology are cystic fibrosis, Tay-Sachs, fragile-X syndrome, and sickle cell anaemia. This type of testing is very complex, individual, and expensive, based on targeting information gained from each parent's DNA. It is not possible or practical to perform this type of testing on every fetus. There is an almost endless list of possible combinations of genes and mutations, so finding one specific disease can be like looking for a needle in a haystack. The field of genetics is rapidly unlocking the keys to finding and detecting these diseases, but we are far from being able to prenatally diagnose them all.

Can you always get accurate results?

With advances in current lab techniques, it is highly unlikely that the result would be inaccurate given that a fetal tissue sample is obtained. Statistics show that the results are accurate 99.4% to 100% of the time. Theoretically, there is always the possibility that the cells that are cultured are maternal cells, not fetal cells (of course, this only applies if the results of the test show female sex chromosomes). This is known as cell contamination, but labs have become very skilled in processing samples and this is no longer a real concern. Every so often, the procedure may fail because the doctor may be unable to acquire a fluid or tissue sample despite making repeated attempts. Factors such as decreased amniotic fluid, a small uterus due to early gestational age, maternal obesity or previous pelvic surgery can hinder the doctor's attempt to gain access to the tissue. If this happens, you can wait a few days and try again. If material is obtained, the lab may sometimes fail to produce a result because the amount of tissue is inadequate or the results are ambiguous. This is slightly more likely to happen with a CVS than an amniocentesis. Very rarely (approximately 1 in 1000 specimens), a sample containing adequate tissue may simply may refuse to grow in the lab. In these cases, a repeat sample can be taken and will almost certainly yield results.

Is there any way to hurry the results?

There are certain circumstances where there is a very high suspicion that the baby could have a chromosomal abnormality. For example, the early ultrasound screening may have shown an abnormally thickened nuchal translucency or other visible anatomical defects. Alternatively, the fetus may have appeared normal, but the integrated blood serum screening showed very high risk results (< 1 in 50). In these cases, your doctor can request preliminary testing be performed on the sample. Faster results are possible using specialized lab techniques, most commonly FISH (fluorescence *in situ* hybridization) and PCR (polymerase chain reaction). These tests only do a basic count and target chromosomes 13, 18, 21, X and Y, as these are the most common places where chromosomal abnormalities occur. FISH testing is the most common way to obtain a preliminary result, often within 48 hours after the lab receives the sample. This is ONLY indicated if there is a very high suspicion that the fetus is abnormal. Preliminary results can be given within 24 to 48 hours. If they are positive, the results are very reliable. Negative results are reassuring but it will still be necessary to wait the 10–14 days for the culture to yield the full karyotyping and analysis. This type of advanced testing is reserved for women who are at exceptionally high risk, since it requires extra time and resources from the workers in the lab to process the sample, making it expensive and impractical for routine use.

If my amniocentesis was normal, do I still need an 18–20 week ultrasound?

The 18–20 week ultrasound is also known as the anatomy scan. During this scan, all visible anatomy from top of the head to the baby's feet is carefully examined to rule out abnormalities such as a cleft lip, problems with the heart, spine, brain, etc. A normal amniocentesis tells us that the fetus has the normal number and structure of chromosomes, but it tells us nothing about the general anatomy, and the baby could still suffer from a range of birth defects. It is true that most babies with abnormal chromosomes will have some anatomical defects, however the vast majority of babies with anatomical defects have normal chromosomes. Therefore, it is still necessary to do an anatomy scan to ensure the fetus has indeed developed as expected. There is other valuable information gained at this scan that can't be gleaned from an amniocentesis or CVS, such as checking the overall growth and size of the baby, viewing the general uterine environment, and probably most importantly, checking the location of the placenta. If the placenta has attached low in the uterus, covering the cervix, it can be carefully monitored during the pregnancy to avoid a potentially disastrous rupture at delivery.

WHICH TESTS ARE RIGHT FOR ME? A DECISION GUIDE

Which statement best describes you?

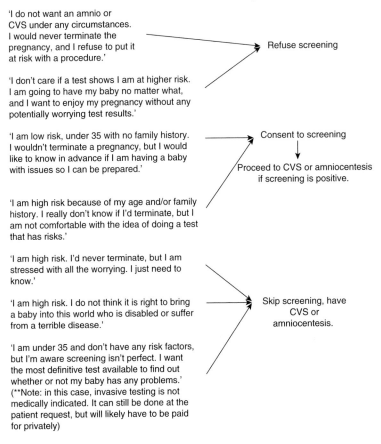

'I do not want an amnio or CVS under any circumstances. I would never terminate the pregnancy, and I refuse to put it at risk with a procedure.'

'I don't care if a test shows I am at higher risk. I am going to have my baby no matter what, and I want to enjoy my pregnancy without any potentially worrying test results.'

Refuse screening

'I am low risk, under 35 with no family history. I wouldn't terminate a pregnancy, but I would like to know in advance if I am having a baby with issues so I can be prepared.'

Consent to screening

Proceed to CVS or amniocentesis if screening is positive.

'I am high risk because of my age and/or family history. I really don't know if I'd terminate, but I am not comfortable with the idea of doing a test that has risks.'

'I am high risk. I'd never terminate, but I am stressed with all the worrying. I just need to know.'

'I am high risk. I do not think it is right to bring a baby into this world who is disabled or suffer from a terrible disease.'

Skip screening, have CVS or amniocentesis.

'I am under 35 and don't have any risk factors, but I'm aware screening isn't perfect. I want the most definitive test available to find out whether or not my baby has any problems.' (**Note: in this case, invasive testing is not medically indicated. It can still be done at the patient request, but will likely have to be paid for privately)

5

General prenatal testing

Key points

- Early prenatal care is essential for ensuring the health and wellbeing of both the mother and the fetus.

- The initial evaluation entails a full physical exam, cervical cytology if necessary, and several blood tests. In addition, a full personal and family medical history will be taken to help your care provider determine which tests should be offered to you.

- Routine visits occur on a regular basis where urine, weight, blood pressure, fetal heart beat, and the growth of the uterus are commonly checked.

- Additional tests that **might** be performed during the pregnancy are glucose testing, Rh antibody status, Group B strep status at 35–36 weeks, and assessment of the cervical readiness for birth towards the end of the pregnancy. You may also be offered fetal fibronectin, non-stress tests (NST), and biophysical profile (BPP) tests.

In the previous chapters, we described the types of testing that can assess the likelihood that a mother is carrying a normal, healthy fetus. We also explained the more invasive testing methods that can be used to obtain a definitive diagnosis if problems are suspected. Every woman is offered screening of her fetus and diagnostic testing when indicated, but not every woman decides to undergo these types of tests. For a variety of personal reasons, many women choose not undergo this testing, especially if voluntarily terminating an abnormal pregnancy is not an option. In this chapter we will address another important aspect of prenatal testing, which is designed to screen and monitor the general health of the mother and the wellbeing of the pregnancy. This type of testing is done with the intent of maximizing the likelihood of a successful birth. It could be argued that this testing is less 'optional' than the screening of the fetus, since refusing some of these tests might put the mother, and therefore the fetus, at risk. However, the woman always has the right to accept or refuse any tests, as long as she has discussed this with her care provider and understands the advantages and disadvantages of her choices.

It is an established fact that women who receive good prenatal care, beginning in the first trimester, will have better outcomes than those who get little or no prenatal care. Early prenatal care allows the care provider to identify medical problems such as diabetes and hypertension (high blood pressure), and to initiate early treatment. Unhealthy behavior, such as poor diet, smoking, drinking, or drug use can also be discussed, giving the provider the opportunity to encourage the mother to modify or eliminate things that may negatively affect pregnancy outcomes.

Initial prenatal evaluation

The initial routine prenatal visit to your care provider is usually one of the longer, more comprehensive assessments that you will have. In addition to discussing your general history, health, and answering any questions you may have, this appointment will often encompass multiple testing procedures. These may include some or all of the following:

- General physical examination and possibly pelvic evaluation.

- Cervical smear (also known as a PAP smear in the USA)

- Prenatal blood tests

- An early ultrasound (described in Chapter 7)

General physical and pelvic evaluation

At this time, a complete physical examination is likely to be performed. This can identify any thyroid or breast abnormalities, as well as other potential health matters. You may also be offered a pelvic exam, especially if you have not had one in a while. This can assist in identifying the location of the pregnancy, the possibility of any pelvic pathology such as abnormal ovarian cysts, and the health and consistency of the cervix (the neck of the womb). If any pelvic abnormalities are suspected, an ultrasound evaluation might be performed.

Cervical cytology

Cervical cytology, also known as a cervical smear (or PAP smear in the USA), examines a sample of cells that are taken from the cervix for changes that may indicate cancerous cells. Your provider may wish to perform this test if you have not had cervical screening, or if it has been 3–5 years since your last test. It is usually performed to allow the early identification of any abnormal cells, ensuring that timely treatment can be instigated. Should the results show any suspicions of abnormality, the cervix will usually be further evaluated by a painless non-invasive microscopic evaluation called colposcopy, which is safe for both mother and fetus. Colposcopy is similar to the cervical smear. The woman lies on her back with her legs apart (or in stirrups) and a colposcope, which is essentially a magnifying device with a bright light, is used to observe the cervix. Some acetic acid (vinegar) may also be used, as it helps to identify any areas that may be abnormal. If any suspicious areas are found, a tiny biopsy may be performed. This involves taking a very small piece of the cervix for analysis, and is harmless to the fetus and only minimally painful for the mother. The biopsy will give important information as to whether any further treatment is necessary. Do not panic if you have an abnormal cervical smear result, as most are caused by infection or inflammation, not cancer.

Initial prenatal blood tests

Many things are checked by the initial blood tests, which means that several tubes of blood are usually taken. While it may seem like a lot of blood, the vials appear larger than they really are, and your body will quickly and easily replenish what was taken without any ill effects for you or the fetus. The tests likely to be run on the blood are as follows:

- Complete blood count: It is important to obtain initial haemoglobin levels to assess whether the pregnant woman is anaemic (low in iron). Should anaemia be present, further testing will often be ordered to identify the cause and to institute treatment, which is often in the form of iron tablets.

- Blood group and Rh factor: These tests identify antibodies than can potentially have adverse effects on the fetus. Should a mother be Rh negative, she will receive additional blood tests and monitoring throughout pregnancy to assess fetal status. If the father of the baby is Rh positive, Rh negative mothers will need an injection of anti-RhD immunoglobulin during the pregnancy (also known as RhoGAM in the USA). This should protect the fetus from any adverse reactions. It will also help prevent the mother from developing antibodies that become permanent in her blood circulation, which could affect any future pregnancies.

◆ Rubella titre: This blood test will identify whether or not you are immune to the German measles virus. If you do not have immunity, you should be vaccinated after delivery. Women who have this test performed prior to conception may be vaccinated in advance of getting pregnant, in order to develop immunity. It is advisable delay conception for three months post-vaccination.

◆ Thyroid function: Thyroid studies are often evaluated, since abnormal thyroid function must be treated during pregnancy to avoid detrimental fetal effects. Low thyroid levels have been linked to poor fetal growth and decreased intelligence, which are easily avoided with proper medication.

Other tests are commonly performed to assess for sexually transmitted diseases such as gonorrhoea and Hepatitis B. It is also advisable to screen for syphilis and HIV; many centres offer the latter test on an opt-out basis. HIV-positive mothers can be intensively treated with antiretroviral drugs during pregnancy to minimize the risk of transmission to the fetus. Screening for other infectious diseases such as parvovirus (also known as Fifths disease), or varicella (chicken pox), may also be performed depending on your history or where you live.

FAQ: 'At my first visit I was asked a lot of questions about not just my OWN family history, but my husband's as well. I don't really know our family histories. Is that information really necessary?' If possible, it is a good idea to prepare for your initial visit by gathering as many details as you can about both you and your partner's family medical history if you don't already know about them. Relevant information that is helpful from **both of you** includes knowing your ethnic origins and any diseases, early deaths, and birth defects that may have affected any of your relatives or ancestors. A family history of mental retardation, blindness, deafness, and so forth are also important to note. Your provider uses this information to help decide which types of genetic blood tests and other screening options are appropriate to offer to you. It can also help him or her determine if a visit to a genetic counsellor is warranted. Of course, sometimes you simply may not be able to obtain accurate or detailed family histories. In these cases, knowing that there is a limited family history will also influence your provider and help him or her to advise you appropriately.

Testing at subsequent and routine interval visits

How often you visit your clinic or provider will vary based on where you live, your circumstances, and your overall health. Generally, regular prenatal visits are likely to occur on a monthly basis in uncomplicated pregnancies up until

28–30 weeks gestation. From 28–36 weeks, visits usually occur at 2 week intervals. Weekly visits may be advised from 36 weeks until birth.

Routine visits are likely to include the following tests:

- **Weight check**: Monitoring a woman's weight allows the provider to assess her nutritional status and to determine whether she may be accumulating extra fluid. If there is evidence of excessive fluid retention (swelling and excessive weight gain), diet and rest may be indicated as well as more frequent obstetrical evaluations.

- **Urine screening**: Your urine will be tested at each prenatal visit, usually for infection, sugar and protein. Abnormal increases in sugar or protein may signify a diabetic state or hypertensive renal disease, both of which necessitate close observation and treatment.

- **Blood pressure**: Blood pressure will be checked at each visit. If it is raised, more frequent monitoring, medications, and additional fetal evaluations may all be indicated.

- **Abdominal examination, including measurement of fundal height**: The fundus is the top of the uterus. While you are lying on your back, your provider uses a tape measure to measure the distance between the pubic bone to the top of your uterus. Measuring the fundal height at each visit allows the provider to assess the fetal growth. Fundal heights should increase throughout pregnancy at an expected rate. If the fundus is higher than expected, this can be indicative of excessive fetal growth or increases in amniotic fluid volume. An unexpectedly small fundal height may signify poor fetal growth or decreases in amniotic fluid volume. Should any abnormalities in fundal growth be observed, further evaluation with ultrasound may be indicated.

- **Fetal heart rate**: Starting at about 8 to 10 weeks, your provider can use a hand-held Doppler device to listen for the baby's heartbeat. These Doppler devices use ultrasound with very low power outputs and are considered very safe. Most units will calculate and display the number of beats per minute. Being able to hear the fetal heart beating is often the highlight of your prenatal visits.

FAQ: 'Should I buy a Doppler heart monitor to use at home?' This is a phenomenon that has become especially common in the USA. If you type in 'fetal heart monitors' on any search engine, you can find countless vendors selling home Doppler monitors. You can buy or rent a monitor, and although they are not cheap, some parents feel it is well worth the investment. There are some advantages to having a home monitor, as it can be tremendously reassuring to hear that little heart beating, especially in the first half of the pregnancy, before you can regularly expect to feel the fetus moving. In the second half of the pregnancy, it can also be a huge relief to be able to do a quick heart check if you haven't felt the fetus move all day or if you are just having a moment of insecurity or worry.

Of course, there are some distinct disadvantages to having this tool, and most midwives and doctors do not encourage parents to bother with it. Finding the heart beat isn't always easy, depending on the position of the fetus, its level of activity, the location of the placenta, and the size of the mother's abdomen. Even seasoned professionals will sometimes struggle, especially early on in the pregnancy. Not finding a heartbeat can induce a lot of unnecessary panic and emergency visits. On the other hand, in the latter part of the pregnancy, if you haven't felt the fetus moving and yet you can hear a heartbeat, you may be falsely reassured. It is important to call your provider if you notice a decrease in fetal movement, even if you are able to hear the heartbeat. Finally, although Doppler ultrasound is considered safe, it is still a form of ultrasound energy and should be used prudently. No one knows whether some adverse effects of ultrasound might be found in future. Checking the heartbeat excessively just doesn't make good sense.

Additional interval testing

AFP testing

AFP stands for alpha-fetoprotein. Around 16 weeks, you will be offered this test. If you consent, your blood will be drawn to test the level of this protein in your blood. Elevated levels of alpha-fetoprotein can indicate that the fetal spine, head, or abdomen are not closed and are leaking fluid into the amniotic cavity. If this blood test proves to be abnormal, this will prompt your provider to order an ultrasound as soon as possible to look for any abdominal, head, or spinal defects. If you are having a triple or a quad screen (explained in Chapter 3) done to screen for a genetically abnormal fetus, this will be part of the test and you will not need to have it done separately. If you had a first tri-mester screen at 10–13 weeks, you will still need to have this tested separately at 16 weeks.

Glucose screening

Women with any risk factors for diabetes, or those who have given birth to large babies in prior pregnancies, will need to be screened for gestational dia-betes. Many providers will screen everyone between 24 and 28 weeks, but this will depend on where you live. Testing consists of consuming a glucose liquid in the clinic, followed 1 hour later by a blood test. If the blood test shows the level of the glucose in the blood is abnormal, an oral glucose tolerance test or 3 hour test may then be ordered to confirm the absence or presence of gestational diabetes. If you are asked to have this test, you will be given specific instructions as to how to prepare, including fasting after bedtime the night before. During the test, you will drink some more glucose liquid, and blood will be drawn hourly to see how your body processes the sugar in the drink. Those found to have gestational diabetes may be treated with diet or medication, depending on circumstances.

Rh antibody testing

As previously mentioned, Rh negative mothers will have blood tests performed during pregnancy to monitor maternal antibody status. Should your antibody screen indicate the presence of Rh antibodies, both mother and fetus will be further evaluated and monitored to minimize the risk of any fetal compromise.

Group B strep cultures

At 35–36 weeks gestation, a group B streptococcus culture might be performed. This is done by taking a gentle swab of the vaginal mucosa and sending the sample to a lab. Group B streptococcus normally lives in the female birth canal; it is harmless and causes no maternal symptoms. However, it can be harmful to the baby, if the baby is infected with Group B streptococcus during a vaginal birth. Some women have these bacteria and some women don't. Its presence is not abnormal, but testing for it in pregnancy allows for prophylactic treatment during labour and birth. A group B strep culture will identify any mother who is a carrier, allowing antibiotics to be administered during labour and minimizing the chance of neonatal infection.

Cervical monitoring

After an initial pelvic examination at the beginning of the pregnancy, there will rarely be any need for internal examinations until much later in the pregnancy, unless for some reason you are at high risk for premature birth. Depending on where you live, you may begin having routine vaginal digital exams from any time after 36 weeks. Your provider will insert their fingers to feel the cervix. This allows the provider to assess the status of the cervix and to detect any dilatation and effacement (also known as thinning) of the cervix. The provider will also be able to identify the presentation of the baby if the abdominal examination findings are unclear (head-down versus breech or transverse), as well as its station (depth in the pelvis). In the UK, pelvic exams are not usually performed towards the end of pregnancy unless clinically indicated, you are past your due date, or you are in labour.

If there is a history of prior cervical surgery (done to diagnose or treat abnormal cervical cells), or a risk of preterm birth is suspected, digital cervical exams may be performed earlier in the pregnancy to look for premature cervical dilatation. Premature cervical dilatation occurs when the cervix starts to open too early; this can eventually lead to a premature birth. The cervix may also be evaluated with serial transvaginal ultrasound assessments. Normally, the cervix should be long and closed until at least the beginning of the third trimester. Any evidence of premature cervical dilatation, or a history of this, may result in the placement of a stitch around the cervix to prevent further dilatation. This is known as a cerclage procedure, and it is usually performed between 16 and 24 weeks. It is usually performed as an outpatient procedure with minimal risks to both mother and baby.

Fetal fibronectin

If there is a history of preterm birth, or if examination and ultrasound evaluations in the second or early third trimesters of pregnancy indicate any evidence of the cervix prematurely dilating (opening), a test may be performed known as fetal fibronectin. A swab is taken of the vagina and cervix which is evaluated to detect the presence of fetal fibronectin. This is a protein produced during pregnancy that acts like a biological glue, attaching the fetal sac to the uterine lining. The presence of fetal fibronectin is a warning that there is a strong possibility of premature labour and birth.

Other potential tests

Problems can sometimes arise during your pregnancy that might lead your provider to suggest additional testing. This is to ensure that the fetus is getting the oxygen and nutrients it needs to thrive inside the uterus. Your provider might want to monitor the fetal heart pattern with a non-stress test (NST). This test is non-invasive and harmless to the fetus. The heartbeat is monitored over a period of time, looking for rises (accelerations) in the heart rate with fetal movement. This is a reassuring sign! Should the heart rate dip (decelerations), it may indicate a potential problem requiring further testing and treatment. If an NST is not as reassuring or reactive as your provider would like to see, it is often because the fetus is just taking a nice deep nap. However, it may prompt your provider to request that you go for an ultrasound known as a biophysical profile (BPP). A full discussion of the BPP and third trimester ultrasound can be found in Chapter 10. Basically, the test consists of evaluating the fetus on multiple levels in an effort to measure its wellbeing. The fetus is examined for muscle tone, practice-breathing, heart rate, general movement, and the amount of amniotic fluid. An abnormal BPP may signal that the fetus is not doing well in the womb. If this happens, further monitoring, hospitalization, and/or early birth may be necessary.

6

Explaining ultrasound

→ Key points

⬦ Ultrasound is an imaging technology that sends sound waves into the body and creates a computer-generated image based on echo return time.

⬦ Ultrasound has been thoroughly investigated and is considered safe for mother and fetus. However, there is a general consensus that it should be reserved for medical purposes, and not used for trivial reasons.

⬦ 2D ultrasound images represent a single slice or plane through the body, and the resultant images are in black, white, and shades of gray.

⬦ 3D images are boxes or sets of 2D images that can be rotated and evaluated in any plane. Using specialized software, the 2D black and white data is manipulated to create the beautiful colour 3D images where you can see the baby's skin and features.

⬦ 3D and 4D ultrasound are essentially the same; however, 3D is a static or still image, 4D is a succession of 3D images over time.

⬦ 3D and 4D ultrasound are not better than standard 2D imaging. While 3D ultrasound is an interesting and sometimes useful technology, 2D is still the standard for diagnostic purposes.

2D ultrasound

Ultrasound images, also known as sonograms, are obtained using ultra high frequency sound waves, in a manner similar to sonar in a submarine or a bat's echo-navigation system. The following is a short, simplified description of how these images are created. The differences and similarities between 2D, 3D, and 4D will also be explained. If you are not technically inclined, or are not interested in how ultrasound works, you can skip to the latter part of this chapter where some of the more common questions concerning ultrasound scans are addressed.

Interpreting the shades of gray

What the colours mean:

Black = Fluid (amniotic fluid, blood, urine)
White = Bone/air
Gray = Soft tissue (fat and muscle)

To create an ultrasound image, the ultrasound probe sends pulses of ultra-high frequency sound into the body. The probe then acts as a listening device, waiting for the returning echoes as the pulses bounce off the tissue and back to the probe. The time it takes for the pulse to return to the probe depends on the density of material it encounters. Different densities have different and predictable return times. Sound travels quickest through liquid, slower through soft tissues like fat or muscle, and ultimately slowest through air, too slow actually to obtain any useful information via ultrasound. Hard bone does not transmit sound but reflects it straight back, leaving a large shadow. This is why ultrasound is not useful for detecting broken bones.

Once the probe has sent sound into the body and measured the return time, software in the ultrasound machine analyzes the data, and gives each pixel or spot on the monitor a shade of gray corresponding to tissue density and depth. This is then updated multiple times per second to make an image which appears 'live' or in real-time.

The ultrasound waves are generated in the probe by piezoelectric crystals, which convert electrical impulses into pulses of sound. These crystals can also convert the returning sound pulses back into electrical signals, which are reconstructed into an image by the machine and its computer. Around 30–40 years ago, when ultrasound first gained acceptance as a medical tool, images were static still-frames in black on white, obtained using an awkward machine with a probe at the end of an unwieldy articulated arm. It yielded images that looked like topographical maps, and offered very limited diagnostic information. Continuing advances in computer processors' ability rapidly to handle and manipulate large amounts of data have led to dramatic improvements in image quality in recent years. Ultrasound images can now be obtained via a hand-held probe in real-time or 'live' imaging, which revolutionizes its diagnostic utility. Computer processing speeds have continued to increase, and software has become ever more sophisticated, leading to continuous improvements in image resolution and the advent of three- and four-dimensional image technology.

The piezoelectric effect

Inside the ultrasound probe (also known as a 'transducer') are piezoelectric crystals, sandwiched between coupling materials which help generate the desired ultrasonic frequencies. When an electrical charge is applied to a piezoelectric crystal, it vibrates to generate mechanical energy (in the form of sound waves). Conversely, the crystals can also transform mechanical energy (sound waves) back into electrical impulses. Piezoelectric crystals housed within ultrasound transducers send ultra-high frequency sound waves out, and receive those waves back after they have echoed off the tissue they encountered. An image is created by the computer using elaborate algorithms.

While 3D and 4D imaging are exciting tools that will be discussed in the next section, the bulk of the images that the sonographer and your doctor will be studying are still made in two dimensions and in black and white. In order

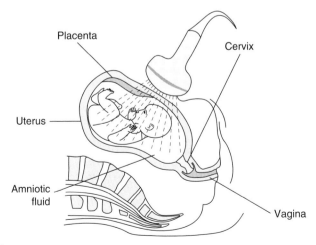

Placenta

Cervix

Uterus

Amniotic
fluid

Vagina

Fig. 6.1

to really appreciate what you are seeing while having your scan, it is helpful to understand a basic idea of cross-sectional anatomy and what it means to think in 2D. When the probe is on the belly, it is not taking a frontal view as in a photograph. Instead, it is taking a thin slice of data directly below the probe from top (mother's skin) to bottom (mother's spine), just as if the probe were a large blade with only the anatomy within the blade visible on the ultrasound monitor. Another helpful way to think in 2D is to picture a loaf of bread, with each single slice representing a single cross sectional image.

Because the probe fits in the hand and is easily rotated, one of the benefits to ultrasound over CT or MRI is the ease with which the probe can be manipulated to take a slice of anatomy in almost any plane. For instance, the probe can be turned to image transversely (imagine a typical slice of bread) or longitudinally (which would yield a slice of the bread cut along the length), or at any axis within 360 degrees (such as cutting the bread diagonally from corner to corner). This is why when you get a great profile view of the baby showing the forehead, nose, lips, and chin, the arms and legs are usually not in the view. Parents are not accustomed to thinking in a single plane, and may be alarmed that their baby 'has no arms' when shown a picture of the fetal profile. Of course the fetus has arms, but if the probe is scanning down the midline of the face, to get a profile including the nose, the arms and legs are on either side of the 'slice,' and are therefore not visible on the screen. Similarly, when we are scanning through the baby's abdomen, you will see a circle. When the focus is on each individual bit of anatomy such as the heart, the area of interest will be isolated and magnified so you aren't going to see the form of the whole baby. Being able to think in a single plane will really help you to understand what you are seeing on the screen.

The importance of gel

When you have an ultrasound scan, you will lie on a bed or exam table next to the ultrasound machine. A water-based gel will be applied on the area to be scanned. The gel acts as a liquid pathway for the sound coming from the probe to travel through into the body, preventing interference from any air that would usually lie between the probe surface and the skin. It also provides a nice friction-free surface for the probe to slide around on comfortably.

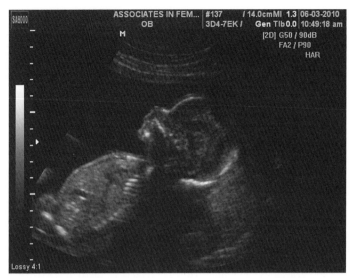

Fig. 6.2 Midline view of 16 week fetus. The arms and legs are not in view because the scan slice is in the midline of the fetus.

3D/4D ultrasound

What's the difference between 3D and 4D?

4D is 3D over **time**

Did you ever draw stick figures on the bottom of the pages of a pad of paper, so that when you flip the pages quickly the figure appears to move? 4D works this way. The effect of motion seen on 4D is created by displaying a rapid succession of still-frame 3D images.

As computer processing speeds and advances in graphics capabilities have increased, the ability for the ultrasound machines to handle, manipulate, and play with huge amounts of data has grown. As a result, the black and white, 2D images that have confused parents for years have given way to beautiful colour images seen on television, websites, magazines, and advertisements. The colour pictures of the baby with the 'skin on' are very exciting for parents, but these don't offer much information diagnostically. That is not to say that 3D is not medically useful (quite the contrary), but there are big differences between the kind of images that a doctor wants to see vs. the attractive images that appeal to parents. A brief explanation of how these images are processed and obtained will clarify why these types of images are not going to replace the traditional black and white images in the foreseeable future.

How 3D images are made

The basic concept in generating a 3D ultrasound image is the same as for a traditional 2D image, described earlier. The probe sends pulses into the body in a single line or plane, and assembles an image from top to bottom based on echo return times. When the 3D imaging function is activated, internal mechanisms within the 3D probe sweep back and forth, instead of acquiring data in a single scan plane from top to bottom. Data is rapidly accumulated along a pre-calibrated horizontal axis so that a box of single planes, called a data set, is acquired. It is because the 3D probe automates the sweeping of the piezoelectric crystals that these probes are so specialized, expensive, and tend to be bulkier and heavier. When a single sweep of data is acquired, there is a 'box' of data stored on the ultrasound unit that can be investigated in **any** plane, including the coronal plane which is unobtainable with traditional 2D imaging. Thinking back to that loaf of bread (explained in the prior section), in 2D we were limited to looking at slices taken across the length, width, or diagonal. In 3D, we can see all those same individual slices but we can also look at slices taken through the center of the bread from top to bottom, virtually cutting the loaf in half like you might if you were making a sandwich, or at any other angle that we choose.

There are many exciting possibilities with 3D, not the least of which is the amount of information that can be reviewed even after the woman has left the building. Post-processing can be done to achieve multiple effects such as slicing out unwanted information, rotating the picture, and changing the background colours. This is similar to editing digital photographs on your home computer to adjust brightness, reduce red-eye, or cut out unwanted objects.

Surface rendering mode

In order to get the photogenic baby pictures that the parents love to see, showing the baby with skin and facial features, the sonographer scans with the 3D probe and uses specific surface rendering modes. This can also be done 'live,' which is known as 4D scanning (the 4th dimension being time).

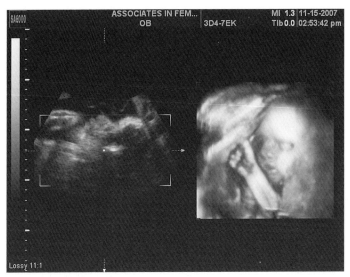

Fig. 6.3 The 3D software manipulates the 2D image on the left to achieve the surface-rendered image on the right.

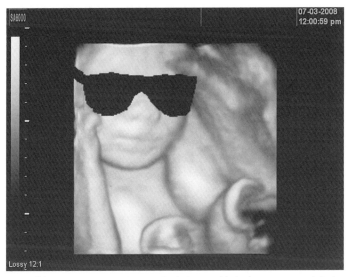

Fig. 6.4 Add some post-processing manipulations and baby becomes a cool dude.

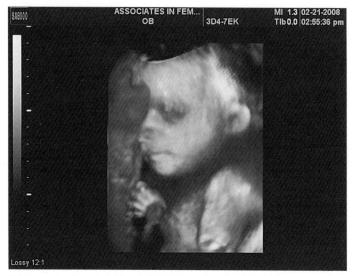

Fig. 6.5 Example of some pitfalls of 3D/4D: The right side of the fetal face and eye is lying against the placenta. No amount of image manipulation will allow a good view of that part of the face. The only way to see it is for the fetus to change position. Also note that part of the hand and arm appears to be missing. The arm is normal but the box of data does not include the forearm and elbow and so the hand appears to be just floating.

Looking at the fetus in 3D and 4D is entertaining, and can truly give you an idea of what the fetus looks like, for instance whether or not the lips are full or what the shape of the face is. Tools in the software usually allow for some manipulation of the image, such as cutting out unwanted areas, and adding text.

A 4D ultrasound scan makes it possible to observe fetal expressions and behaviour, from grimaces to smiles, sucking and licking movements, and limb motion, such as all babies display after birth. However, the sonographer's ability to get good pictures of the face is completely dependent on the fetal position. The ultrasound machine requires a 'window' or space of fluid in front of the face to construct a good surface rendered view. If the arms, placenta, or uterine wall are lying directly against the face, this will block some or all of the view.

Are 3D/4D images medically useful?

As attractive as the surface-rendered images can be, they will not replace black and white, 2D images. Putting skin on the baby defeats the purpose of what the sonographer is trying to do medically. If you hurt your knee, the doctor needs to do more than just look at it. He/she uses an X-ray or MRI to see

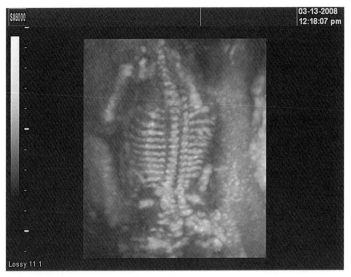

Fig. 6.6 Another post-processing feature: 'X-ray mode' (as opposed to surface rendering) of the spine and ribs.

beyond the skin to the ligaments and bones inside. Similarly, with prenatal ultrasound, doctors need to see beyond the surface of the fetus to evaluate the internal structures. However, the ability of 3D technology to allow views of anatomy in multiple planes has much to offer obstetrics and will likely drive many changes and advancements in the field in the future. For example, multiple individual images of the fetal heart and each organ are painstakingly taken with 2D imaging, which can take a lot of time to complete. Once providers become more comfortable scanning fetuses using the multiplanar 3D (saving boxes of data to be reviewed later), a single pass of the probe from the fetal abdomen up to the neck can be saved and can yield all the information needed on all the internal structures. The same can be done for the head, heart, spine, and so on, reducing the overall scan time from 30–45 minutes to just a few. Even surface rendering has some medical uses, and is especially helpful to clarify the extent or severity of external defects such as a cleft lip or club foot. However, the reality of providing quality obstetrical ultrasound today is that 3D/4D ultrasound is still more of a perk than a necessity. The traditional 2D images can provide all the information needed to evaluate a pregnancy properly.

FAQ: 'Why did they tell me to drink lots of water when I made my ultrasound appointment?' Ultrasound travels beautifully through fluid, allowing structures to be seen behind it with greater clarity and resolution.

A full bladder conveniently lies above the uterus and cervix, pushing bowel out of the way and providing a clear window to see into the uterus. Bowel always contains air, which interferes with looking at anything behind it, so a full bladder can really make a big difference in obtaining quality images. However, as your uterus grows, it eventually extends beyond even the fullest bladder, so it is not as important in the 2nd and 3rd trimesters to be uncomfortably full. Fortunately, the amniotic fluid surrounding the fetus will usually provide enough of a window to see what is needed.

FAQ: 'Is ultrasound safe?' In over 40 years of practice and research, there have been no proven cases of harm caused by the use of medical ultrasound at normal diagnostic frequencies. However, remember that ultrasound involves sending high frequency sound waves into the body, which pass through and are bounced off the maternal tissues and the fetus. These high frequency waves have energy, and at extreme intensities (above those normally used for diagnostic imaging) they have been shown in laboratory conditions to heat tissue and induce cavitation, or the formation of microbubbles. All ultrasound machines manufactured for use in medical practice have preset controls built into the units that should prevent them from emitting dangerously high power outputs and intensities, but the fact that ultrasound does transmit energy means it should be treated with respect. There is likely no harm in having multiple scans during a pregnancy performed by qualified medical personnel, who will ensure the power outputs are in the safe range. However, all medical governing bodies in all countries agree that it is a bad idea to use ultrasound in a non-medical setting for the purpose of personal entertainment.

FAQ: 'Can the baby hear the ultrasound?' We hear this question a lot and have seen strange stories on the internet about this. People have assumed that because the fetus often has its hands up by the head and ears, it is trying to shield itself from the 'noise'. This is absolutely false. The range of audible sound for human beings includes sound waves that have a range between 20 and 20,000Hz (20–20KHz). In contrast, diagnostic ultrasound has wavelengths that range from approximately 3 **million** to 8 **million** Hz (3–8MHz). Not even dogs can hear in this range. The fetus certainly isn't hearing it either. Sometimes the ultrasound probe can and does emit an audible hum or high ringing sound perceptible to adult, and possibly fetal, ears; this is a harmless side effect of scatter of the frequencies the probe is emitting.

FAQ: 'Does 3D/4D increase ultrasound exposure?' 3D/4D does not apply any additional exposure to ultrasound energy than traditional 2D. 3D/4D images are made by using the exact same 2D waves, the difference lies in how the internal computer manipulates the sound data obtained.

Medical advantages of 3D vs. 2D

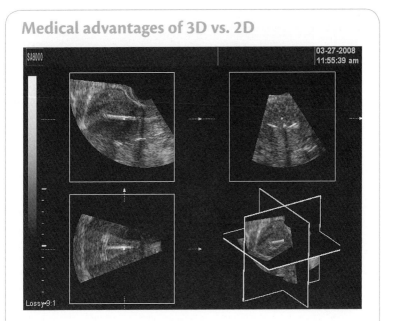

Can you guess what this is? (Hint: this is a non-pregnant woman)

Using 3D ultrasound imaging allows for views of anatomy never before obtainable on traditional 2D imaging. The above image shows how 3D is actually multiple planes of 2D, with the upper left image a long view (from head to toe) of a non-pregnant uterus, the upper right image a transverse (from hip to hip)view, both of which are obtainable with traditional real-time 2D scanning. Because a whole box of data is saved in the machine when the sonographer utilizes the 3D options, a look can be taken at that third plane (lower left image), which is anatomically impossible to obtain when scanning hands-on and live. These 3 planes are illustrated by the coloured square boxes on the lower right image, the dissecting box (representing the coronal plane) being completely unique to 3D. The various planes can each be moved up or down, and rotated on multiple axes, allowing for complete evaluation of the volume box. Skillful manipulation of the data allows us to get this beautiful view of an IUD (see below) showing perfect placement within the triangular-shaped endometrial cavity of the uterus.

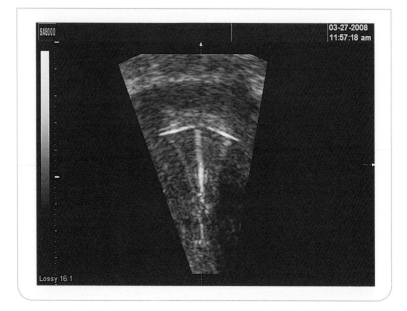

7

Early first trimester ultrasound

> ## ➲ Key points
>
> ◆ Ultrasound in the early first trimester can detect a fetal heartbeat as early as 6 weeks from the first day of the last menstrual period (LMP).
>
> ◆ Most of the time, if you have an early ultrasound scan it will be performed transvaginally.
>
> ◆ The main purpose of an early first trimester scan is to establish the viability, location, dates, and number of embryos.

The transvaginal ultrasound

Scans in the first trimester can sometimes be done abdominally (when the probe is placed on the skin below the navel), but most of the time, better images are obtained using a vaginal approach. Many women are aware of the 'probe' or 'wand' used, having had this type of scan previously for gynaecological reasons, or having heard about it from family and friends. Basically, the transducer is shaped like a tampon and is covered with a condom-like protective cover. Gel or lubricant is applied to the end of the covered probe, and the probe is then inserted into the vagina with minimal discomfort. The transvaginal probe has much higher resolution than the abdominal scanner; therefore it is able to visualize smaller structures with much greater detail. Because of this excellent resolution, a heartbeat is visible in an embryo as tiny as 3 mm, corresponding to 6 weeks from the last menstrual period (LMP). The probe only enters the vaginal canal, does not disturb the cervix or the uterus, and is perfectly safe even if you are experiencing some bleeding or cramping. Another advantage to the transvaginal exam is that it does not require an uncomfortably full bladder, which would be necessary if the scan were to be done through the abdomen.

Smaller structures are better visualized transvaginally, but the trade-off for the increased resolution is a smaller field of view. As with a microscope, things that are close can be seen very well, but anything further away is a blur. By approximately 12 weeks gestation, the uterus and fetus have grown larger and have moved up towards the mother's navel, beyond the visual reach of the vaginal probe. As a result, most ultrasound scanning after 10–12 weeks will be done transabdominally.

Viability

In general, 1 in 4 to 1 in 5 pregnancies end in miscarriage. Those odds get even worse the older you get. While this may sound like an exaggerated number, early miscarriages are unfortunately all too common. Only about one generation ago, before the advent of home pregnancy tests that can detect pregnancy several days **before** the first missed period, women would have had to wait for at least 2 missed periods before they would suspect or test for pregnancy. This meant that by the time their pregnancy was confirmed, they were practically finished with the first trimester. If bleeding began before then, they often assumed that they must have been 'late', skipped a period, or had a false alarm. Many of these cases were likely to have been early miscarriages, but women were spared the disappointment and heartache of knowing that for sure.

Things are very different now. Most women have reliably confirmed their pregnancy within a day or two of their missed period, thanks to the outstanding accuracy of home pregnancy tests. Some tests can even detect pregnancy up to 4 days **before** a missed period. This has definite advantages. Women can make early lifestyle changes that will benefit the pregnancy, such as giving up drinking alcohol, stopping smoking, and beginning a prenatal vitamin and folic acid regimen. However, such early detection also incurs a deep sense of loss and disappointment if the pregnancy doesn't progress. All too often, an embryo simply doesn't develop, or stops developing very early in the process. So many things have to go right in order for something as complex as a human to develop; the cascade of various hormones needed to produce an egg to be fertilized, proper implantation in a good place in the uterus, the division of 2 cells into millions of cells, organizing and specializing to become brain, bone, spine, organs, limbs, and so on. If something is going to go wrong with an embryo's development, it usually happens in these initial stages. What many people don't realize is that the gestational sac grows independently of whether or not there is an actual live embryo developing. The gestational sac is the place where the baby is supposed to be growing within the uterus. The chorionic villi, which comprise the early forming placenta, continue to divide and grow, increasing in size and number as if there were an embryo inside, even if the sac is empty. The uterus will continue to enlarge. The pregnancy hormones found in the blood tests and urine will still be present and rising, although perhaps not at an optimal rate (see Chapter 1, Diagnosing Pregnancy). The woman will 'feel' pregnant, nauseous with sore breasts and other pregnancy symptoms. Usually by 7–9 weeks, but sometimes even as late as 12 weeks, the body finally recognizes that there is no live embryo, and bleeding will start. These pregnancies are known as blighted ova or missed abortions, and they comprise the bulk of early miscarriages.

Identifying a good pregnancy versus a blighted one is the main reason for doing an early first trimester ultrasound. It will prove that an embryo has in fact developed, and that it has a heartbeat. Once the heartbeat is detected (which can be as early as 6–6.5 weeks from the LMP), we know that the chance of a miscarriage now drops from the statistical 20–25% to less than 5%. The tradition of waiting until 12 weeks to make 'the announcement' is rooted in those days before we were able to see what was happening inside the uterus. Therefore, if you see a heartbeat on your early ultrasound, you can feel as confident that things are going to go well as your mother did when she hit the 12-week mark and her doctor could finally hear the heart beat. Of course, if you have a history of genetic defects, multiple losses, or other complicating risk factors, your potential for a problem might still be higher. Even so, the greatest and most reassuring hurdle in any pregnancy is the development of a heartbeat.

FAQ: 'When is it safe to announce our pregnancy?' This is a very personal decision, dependent upon your own privacy needs. Traditionally, many people felt it necessary to keep it to themselves throughout the entire first trimester for fear of an early miscarriage. As discussed, however, barring any unusual risk factors, if there is a fetal heartbeat at 7 or 8 weeks, your likelihood of a miscarriage is not significantly different than it would be if you wait until 12 weeks to announce it to friends and family. On the other hand, there are many parents who still prefer to keep it to themselves until the results of the 12 week genetic screening tests are in. This is especially reasonable if you are uncomfortable with the implications of pursuing invasive testing and possible termination of the pregnancy should you get abnormal results.

Timeline for visualizing structures

4.5–5 weeks from LMP: Gestational sac can be seen in the uterus.

5–6 weeks from LMP: Yolk sac should be visualized within the gestational sac.

6–6.5 weeks from LMP: An embryo with a visible heartbeat should be seen.

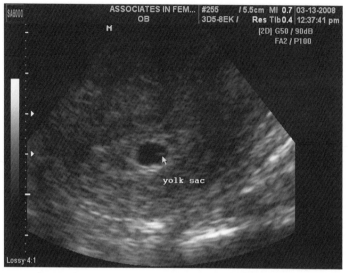

Fig. 7.1 Early **5 week** pregnancy. The embryo is not visible yet, but the dark circle of the gestational sac (early amniotic cavity) and the yolk sac inside (arrow) can be seen. The yolk sac is a bubble of nutrients that nourishes the developing embryo until the placenta takes over that task by the end of the first trimester.

FAQ: 'How early can we see or hear the heartbeat?' If an embryo can be seen, a heartbeat should be detected. The earliest the embryo can be visible is when it is about 2.5–3 mm, or about 6 weeks from the LMP. Often, it is the small pulsing movement that enables sonographers to find the tiny embryo when it is 'hiding' at the edge of the sac or against the uterine wall.

FAQ: 'Does the baby have a good heartbeat?' Any heart beat is usually a good sign. The only time a heartbeat is of concern is if it is very early in the pregnancy (less than 8 weeks) and the heart rate is low, around 80–100 bpm (beats per minute). This can mean that we are detecting motion driven by the mother's circulation, not true embryonic heart motion. When the embryo's heartbeat is measured early, at around 6 weeks, rates as low as 110–120 bpm are normal. By 7–8 weeks, the fetal heart rate should have accelerated to 120–160 bpm, where it will remain for the rest of the pregnancy. Fluctuations in heart rate from one visit to the next or even one minute to the next are not a cause for concern and are actually normal.

FAQ: 'My baby's heart rate is 160bpm. Isn't that too high?' A heart rate that high is completely normal. Again, fetal heart rates are expected to range from 120–160 bpm, and may rise higher towards the end of the pregnancy.

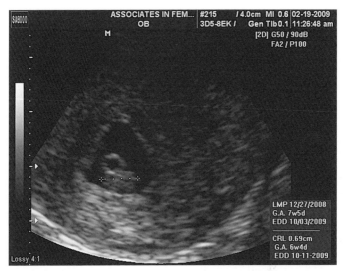

Fig. 7.2 1 week later, you can now see that the gestational sac (dark area) appears larger and there is a 7 mm embryo, corresponding with **6 weeks + 4 days**. Sitting directly above the embryo is the yolk sac. This measurement shows that there is an 8 day discrepancy between the LMP date and the actual gestation date. Based on this early scan, the doctor may consider adjusting the due date.

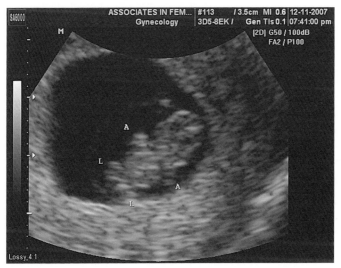

Fig. 7.3 8 weeks. A recognizable head versus body is now evident, as well as limb buds. The embryo now measures 2 cm or 0.75 inches.

Typically, the smaller the creature, the faster the heart beat. A hummingbird, for example, has a heart rate of up to 1,260 bpm, a mouse is around 500 bpm, and an adult human is 70 bpm, while an elephant is slower at 28 bpm. In general, heart rate is dependent on the length of the route that the blood has to flow in order to make one complete circuit. So, being smaller in size, a fetus, baby, or child will all have a faster resting heart rate than an adult.

FAQ: 'What happens if I miscarry?' Should you experience significant bleeding after a positive pregnancy test, you may have had a miscarriage. An ultrasound can show if there is any retained tissue in the uterus. If so, a surgical procedure known as a D&C (dilatation and curettage) may be necessary. A D&C is a simple and quick procedure where the cervix is dilated under anaesthesia and a scraping of the uterine cavity is performed. Usually this is an outpatient procedure and you will be able to go home on the same day. In some cases, there may not be any bleeding at all, but ultrasounds may show that there is not a live embryo or that the gestational sac is empty. You and your doctor may decide to do a D&C, or you may choose to wait and see if the pregnancy passes spontaneously and completely on its own.

Dates

Another benefit to an early ultrasound is the opportunity to date the pregnancy with the greatest degree of accuracy. The measurement of the fetus from crown to rump can accurately determine the age of the embryo to within a few days. The correlation between this measurement and the pregnancy date has been well researched, and the long-established tables are programmed into the software of the ultrasound machine. Up to 8 weeks, there is not a lot of variability in size from embryo to embryo, and the dating is accurate to within 4 or 5 days. With every passing week of the pregnancy, dating becomes less accurate via fetal measurements since individual variations in genetics, size, and prenatal environment begin to be expressed. For example, a normal healthy baby can be born at a legitimate 40 weeks, right on its due date, and weigh anywhere from 6 pounds to 10 pounds (or more). That doesn't mean the baby is older or younger, normal or abnormal. It is simply demonstrating an individual tendency to be petite versus large, short versus tall, etc.

In the early ultrasound, if the embryo measures within the same week as expected by the woman's last menstrual period (LMP), then the due date based on the LMP will be confirmed. If, however, there is a discrepancy of more than 5 to 7 days, your provider may adjust your due date, basing it on the earliest scan and crown-rump length. The LMP due date is usually on target if the woman has a regular 28 day cycle, and if ovulation and fertilization occurred around day 14. Since many women have longer or shorter cycles, ultrasound dating allows for greater confidence in the accuracy of establishing a valid due date. Only 5% of babies are actually born exactly on their due dates. However, it is important to establish a 'due date,' since most prenatal tests are dependent on being performed at specific times during the pregnancy. Of course, if you go beyond your due date, your provider will want to know exactly when being late is getting *too* late.

Location

Another aspect of pregnancy that the early scan will verify is that the gestational sac is located **in** the uterus where it belongs. If the pregnancy does not implant inside the uterine cavity, but rather grows in the fallopian tubes or pelvis, it is known as an ectopic pregnancy. Fortunately, this is uncommon, occurring in approximately 2% of all pregnancies. It is important to rule this out as early as possible, because an ectopic pregnancy can have serious, even fatal consequences for the mother if left undiagnosed.

Number

Two or more gestations can be reliably diagnosed at this early point in the pregnancy. Twins occur in approximately 2–5% of all pregnancies. Most twins or multiples are fraternal (also known as non-identical), meaning that each one is a unique and separate fertilized egg which implants in its own place in the uterus. Identical twinning is quite rare compared to fraternal (non-identical) twinning, occurring in approximately 0.2% of all pregnancies and only 8% of all twin pregnancies. When a single embryo splits into two to become identical twins, the ideal scenario is for it to happen early in the development so that each embryo has its own gestational sac and placenta, mimicking the set-up for all fraternal (non-identical) twins. A less ideal situation occurs if the egg splits later, with the twins sharing a placenta, but each having their own yolk sac and amniotic sac. If they split even later, they may share a placenta **and** an amniotic sac, and splits even later than that can be conjoined. All of these cases, especially the latter two, are at very high risk for complications and would be very carefully monitored.

Identifying twins or multiples with ultrasound is very easy and is very unlikely to be missed with today's technology. It is possible to know that there are twins even before the embryos are visible, especially with fraternal (non-identical) twins, as each one will have its own separate gestational sac and yolk sac. Patients often wonder if it is possible to miss a twin, and almost everyone seems to be able to recount a story where there was a surprise twin at delivery, but in this day and age such a scenario is tremendously unlikely.

FAQ: 'Can you always tell identical versus fraternal twins?' Sometimes, it is possible to know early on with certainty that the two fetuses are identical

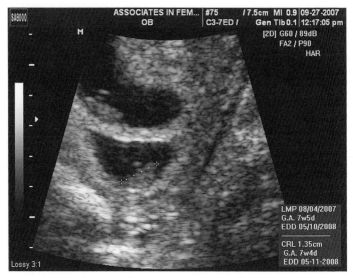

Fig. 7.4 Early 7.5 week twins with two separate gestational sacs, each containing an embryo and yolk sac. These could be either fraternal or identical, although fraternal twins are more common and therefore more likely.

twins if they are sharing an amniotic sac or placenta. Identical twins come from the *same* fertilized egg, which splits into two embryos. In contrast, fraternal twins are *two completely separate* fertilized eggs. With fraternal (non-identical) twins, in the first trimester you will always see two independent gestational sacs, each with its own placenta and each containing a yolk sac and embryo as seen in Fig. 7.6. However, you can also see this with identical twins if they split very early. Identical twins always are the same sex, so if one is a boy and the other a girl, then there is no question - they must be non-identical. On the other hand, if you have twins in separate sacs with separate placentas and they are the same sex, then you won't know whether or not they are identical until after birth. Even after birth, DNA testing may be necessary to be definitive. Of course, they're *probably* fraternal (non-identical) since that is the more common type of twinning, but you won't know for sure until they are born.

FAQ: 'They found a cyst on my ovary on my early ultrasound. Should I be concerned?' Ovarian cysts are commonly seen with early ultrasound evaluations. In fact, an ovarian cyst is essential for ovulation and maintaining the pregnancy as it begins to grow. The cyst is known as a corpus luteum. It secretes progesterone and estrogens, which prime and plump the endometrial lining, allowing the early pregnancy to implant and develop. By the end of the first trimester, the placenta takes over hormone production, and the cyst

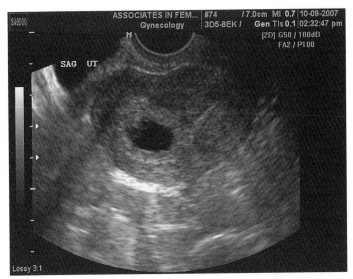

Fig. 7.5 Early 5 week transvaginal view. Note the two yolk sacs (two bubbles) lying within the single gestational sac. Even this early into the pregnancy, we already know this is a case of identical twinning.

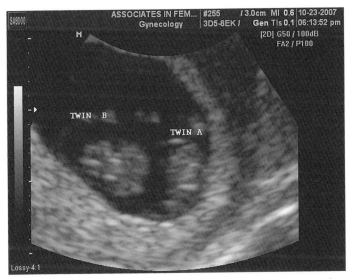

Fig. 7.6 The same identical twins, 2 weeks later. Now, we can see two separate embryos, each with its own amniotic sac (the faintly visible bubble) seen around each embryo.

will be reabsorbed and disappear. Corpus luteal cysts can measure up to 3 cm or 1.5 inches and have a typically simple, round appearance. They will not require any further attention. Occasionally, these cysts will not appear completely simple and can contain some internal debris or septations. In that case, the size and ultrasound characteristics of the cyst will determine if your provider will request you to return for follow up ultrasounds. If the cyst does not resolve after a period of time or if it develops a suspicious appearance, it will be closely monitored throughout the pregnancy. Rarely, surgical intervention may be necessary. Most often, this is not the case and the cyst completely resolves on its own.

8

The nuchal translucency scan: 11–13 weeks

Key points

- By 12 weeks, the embryo has developed into a recognizably human fetus with most of the anatomy complete. From this point onwards, it only has to grow and mature.

- The primary purpose of the 12 week scan is to obtain a nuchal translucency (NT) measurement, an integral part of first trimester screening. Some places might also include the fetal nasal bone and other parameters into the screening.

- The NT is small collection of fluid that lies just under the skin at the fetal neck. It is considered thickened if it is greater than 3 mm, and this indicates that the fetus is at higher risk for a chromosomal abnormality.

- If the fetus is found to be chromosomally normal, but has a thickened NT, careful monitoring will be necessary, because these fetuses are at higher risk for anatomical abnormalities or syndromes. However, in the majority of cases, the fetus is still likely to be normal.

- An evaluation of the fetal anatomy is also commonly performed at this scan, although this is limited by the small size of the structures.

In the early first trimester ultrasound, the embryo looked like a seahorse or gummy bear. Since it isn't recognizably human yet, one could imagine it growing into anything from a polar bear to a beluga whale. By 12 weeks, the embryo has grown into an easily recognizable, miniature human being, approximately 8 cm or 2.5 inches long, with arms, legs, fingers, organs, brain, and skull. Parents are almost always surprised by how well they can see the fetus and by how active it is. During the course of an average examination, most fetuses will spend at least some time moving and flexing.

The 12 week scan is part of a relatively recent development in first trimester screening, aimed at finding those fetuses that are at higher risk for being chromosomally abnormal. There are different names for the testing such as 'first trimester screen', 'ultra-screen', or 'nuchal translucency ultrasound,' depending on the laboratory where the test is performed. This testing was pioneered in the UK, led by Kypros Nicolaides, MD and the Fetal Medicine Foundation, and is now a routine standard of care in most countries. A huge amount of data has been amassed regarding its accuracy and efficacy in finding those fetuses that are at higher risk for genetic abnormalities, of which Down's syndrome is the most commonly known. As discussed in Chapter 3, this screening is multi-faceted, combining measurements obtained by ultrasound with maternal blood sampling. The purpose of the ultrasound portion is to obtain a measurement of a tiny sliver of fluid that lies just under the skin behind the neck known as the nuchal translucency (NT). The sonographer needs additional training and certification to perform this very specialized scan. The general cut-off for a normal versus suspicious measurement of the NT is 3 mm. Any measurement 3 mm. or greater gives cause for concern and further testing. Fetuses with an increased measurement are typically at risk for Down's Syndrome or other chromosomal abnormalities. It is not completely understood why the NT might be thicker in fetuses with abnormal chromosomes, but it has been found that the critical window of time to obtain the measurement is between 10.5 and 13 weeks. Interestingly, beyond 13 weeks, the nuchal thickness may revert to normal even if the fetus is abnormal. If the NT is greater than 3 mm, further testing may show that the chromosomes are indeed normal. However, these fetuses need close follow-up, since they are more likely to have anatomical defects such as heart abnormalities, cystic hygroma (cystic neck mass), or other structural problems. It is important to note that in the majority of cases where there is a thickened NT, the fetus is still very likely to be chromosomally and anatomically normal. However, it is a sign that invasive testing should be offered, and some additional ultrasound scanning should be performed as the pregnancy progresses.

As explained in Chapter 3, in order to obtain final results for the first trimester screening, the NT measurement taken by the sonographer on ultrasound is combined with lab results on the blood sample taken from the mother. The lab identifies the levels of a group of specific chemical markers in the maternal blood, factors in the NT measurement, age of the mother, and sometimes a measurement of the nasal bone (depending on where you have the test) and is able to come up with a statistical risk analysis of the likelihood that fetus might suffer from a chromosomal abnormality. Because the test does not rely on the ultrasound measurements alone, even after a normal ultrasound, the woman

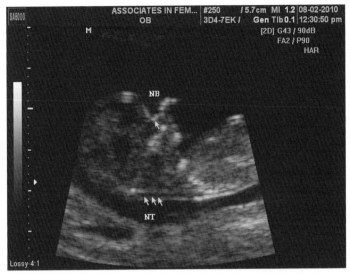

Fig. 8.1 Nuchal translucency (NT) and nasal bone (NB).The NT is the tiny stripe of fluid lying just under the skin at the back of the neck that is measured at the 12-week scan. This measurement needs to be accurate to the nearest 0.01cm, so it needs to be performed by a specially trained and NT certified sonographer or sonologist with quality equipment. Note: the white dots by the nose are the fingers. Very often, the hands are seen by the head and face.

may still get a call a few days later that the fetus was found to be higher risk and further testing with chorionic villus sampling (CVS) or amniocentesis might be indicated. While it may be reassuring to get an NT measurement below 3 mm and normal blood results, it is still not a guarantee of zero risk. First trimester screening will accurately flag abnormal fetuses approximately 90–94% of the time (thus missing around 6–10% of abnormal babies), whereas amniocentesis or CVS provides 100% assurance.

Other structures evaluated in a typical 12 week scan

Most of the time, the NT scan is done transabdominally. Occasionally, for various reasons such as maternal size or fetal position, a transvaginal ultrasound might be performed. At this scan, in addition to the NT measurement, the fetus will be measured from crown to rump, the heart rate will be documented, and basic anatomical structures such as the hemispheres in the brain, the limbs, abdominal wall, stomach, and bladder will be observed. The scan will also verify that the amniotic fluid volume, placenta, uterus, and maternal ovaries look normal. Documentation of the presence of the fetal nasal bone might also be done at this scan although it is not done everywhere. Eventually, nasal bone measurements might be incorporated into the first trimester screening globally, since there is data to support that the absence or shortening of the nasal bone can be a sign of an abnormal fetus. At present, the data and validity of using the nasal bone as well as other potential markers for abnormalities is still being investigated. Ongoing research and the constant drive towards improving screening detection rates may mean that the screening test you receive may differ slightly from region to region and year to year.

FAQ: 'Can the sex be determined at this time?' It's not impossible to tell the sex at the 12 week scan; however, it can be a gamble and you certainly shouldn't regard an answer based on this early scan as definitive. Both boys and girls have external genitalia at this point, so it would be very easy to make an incorrect prediction.

In order to attempt a prediction at this early stage, a midline slice in 2D black/white imaging is taken to look at the direction of the phallus in relation to the fetal sacrum. If it appears to extend perpendicular to the sacrum, then it's likely to be a boy, whereas if it runs parallel, then it's probably a girl.

Very often, the phallus does not seem to be committed to running parallel or perpendicular, but instead lies somewhere in the middle. This seems to happen more often than not, so don't count on finding out the baby's sex at the 12 week scan. By 16 weeks, the genitalia have usually developed into easily

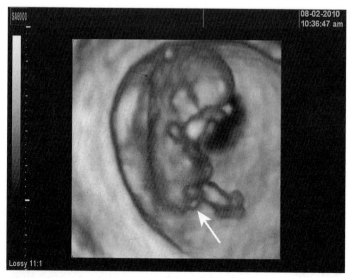

Fig. 8.2 11 wk 3D view of embryo showing external phallus. This fetus turned out to be a girl!

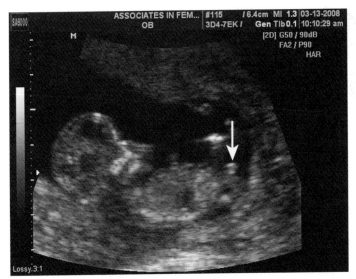

Fig. 8.3 Phallus appears perpendicular, typical for a boy.

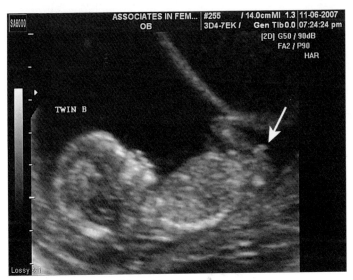

Fig. 8.4 Parallel phallus, typical for a girl.

recognizable male or female features. However, unless you have an amniocentesis at 16 weeks, the next scan you will typically get is the anatomy scan at around 18 to 20 weeks, at which point the gender can almost always be confidently revealed.

FAQ: 'If my 12 week ultrasound and screening results are normal, do I still need a 20 week scan?' At 12 weeks, most of the anatomy is fully developed and can be completely evaluated with close ultrasonic examination. However, as you can imagine, the anatomy is tiny and subtle defects can be missed. There are also changes in the brain and details within the heart, face, body, and limbs that cannot be predicted or fully observed yet. A full examination at approximately 20 weeks is needed to ensure that all has indeed developed normally. Even if you prove normal chromosomes with a CVS or amniocentesis that does not guarantee that all the anatomy is normal. Babies can be born with normal chromosomes yet still suffer a myriad of physical abnormalities or syndromes. 12 weeks is also too early to tell whether or not the placenta is in a safe location for vaginal birth, and whether or not the amniotic fluid and overall growth is within expected parameters.

9

The anatomy scan: 18–20 weeks

➔ Key points

- The anatomy scan is the most extensive ultrasonic examination of the fetus in the pregnancy, and is usually performed between 18 and 22 weeks.

- All visible anatomy, from the fetal head and brain to the feet, is carefully evaluated and documented.

- Fetal growth, amniotic fluid, the uterus, and the placenta are also evaluated.

- The fetal gender can almost always be reliably revealed at this examination if the mother so chooses.

- The anatomy ultrasound is an abdominal scan. Transvaginal scanning in the 2nd trimester is usually only performed if there is risk of pre-term birth.

Advantages of routine anatomy scanning

The anatomy scan, also known as an anatomic survey or anomaly scan, is the most extensive ultrasound you are likely to have, and is the one most people are referring to when they think about ultrasound in pregnancy. It is probably most notable for being the time when the sex can be reliably revealed, in areas where informing the parents of their child's gender is permitted within practice guidelines. There has been debate as to whether this test should be performed routinely in every pregnancy, especially in cases where pregnancy termination is not an option. Doctors and midwives have no problem respecting a choice to refuse the genetic screening earlier in the pregnancy, but they might try to talk you out of refusing the anatomy scan. Studies consistently show that infant mortality rates decrease in settings where anatomy scans have been performed. Additionally, maternal complications are decreased, especially in cases where the placenta is improperly implanted. It is no surprise that if a problem or serious defect is found in the fetus, the baby has a better chance for survival and successful correction if it is detected <u>before</u> birth. Prenatal detection allows parents and providers to plan for the birth to take place in a hospital that is equipped to care for a sick newborn, and allows the medical team to prepare a strategy for special needs in advance. For instance, if your baby has a heart defect, delivering in a small county clinic as opposed to a specialist hospital staffed with paediatric cardiologists, ready to move in with the proper equipment in the delivery room, can literally mean the difference between life and death.

Most major defects will have to wait until birth to be treated. However, there are some temporary interventions that can be performed in utero (while the baby is still in the womb) that can dramatically affect the overall outcome. Doctors can operate on the fetus through a small hole in the uterus using a thin telescopic surgical tool known as a fetoscope. For example, if the fetal kidneys or bladder are blocked, shunts or tubes can be placed to allow the trapped fluid to drain into the amniotic sac. This can prevent the kidneys or bladder from being overdistended and destroyed. Most of these measures are just temporary fixes and surgery will still be required after birth, but they can definitely improve the prognosis.

There may be less dramatic information obtained at this scan that you reasonably may not wish to know, the gender being the most obvious. Gender is not going to be divulged unless you ask, but there may be other things such as the finding of soft markers. Soft markers are subtle, non-definitive and usually harmless physical signs that the baby might have Down's syndrome. These are discussed more fully later in this chapter, but if they are found, you might be told that your baby has a higher risk of Down's syndrome and offered invasive testing. Some people have no interest in consenting to an invasive test that carries a risk of miscarriage, even if there is a possibility that the fetus has Down's syndrome. They may feel comfortable progressing with a pregnancy even if there are problems, since termination of a pregnancy is not a personal option. Others prefer not to know whether they are low, intermediate, or high risk, and will address whatever challenges they may have to face in due course. If this applies to you, it is important to speak openly with your doctor or midwife and communicate your wishes before your scan.

The anatomy ultrasound scan almost always takes much longer than any other scan in the pregnancy, usually lasting 30–45 minutes, occasionally more. Since there is so much that needs to be evaluated and documented on this scan, examination time is dependent on fetal position and cooperation. This is analogous to bringing a toddler to a portrait studio and getting them to sit calmly and smile. If the fetus is being uncooperative, the mother may be asked to roll on one side or the other, give a gentle jiggle on her belly, or take a short walk. Often, patience is the only thing that works: eventually the fetus will roll over. If the baby still isn't in a good position, the woman may be asked to sit in the waiting room to try again later, or to return to try again on another day.

The anatomy scan is also time-consuming because the entire fetal anatomy is evaluated and documented. While the idea of finding out the sex is what often makes this scan so eagerly anticipated, it is important not to underestimate the medical value of this examination. Most of the other ultrasounds are usually comprised of 8 to 12 images that become part of the patient's stored medical file. In contrast, at this scan there are dozens of required images that need to be taken, often 40 to 50 or more end up getting permanently stored. Each piece of anatomy or area of interest will be targeted in specific cross sections or slices (as explained earlier in Chapter 6, the '2D Ultrasound' section). These can look very confusing and uninteresting to the untrained audience.

Targeted anatomy at 20 Week Scan:

- Head and brain
- Face, lips, and eyes
- Spine
- Heart
- Diaphragm
- Stomach
- Bladder
- Kidneys
- Umbilical cord
- Limbs
- Hands and feet

- Placenta

- Amniotic fluid

- Maternal cervix

Even though it may take a while, each and every picture that is taken is targeted to rule out a variety of specific anomalies.

Images obtained at the anatomy scan

Head and Brain: Cross-sections of the skull and brain at the level of the midbrain are taken and measured. The image is not of the 'top' of the head, but comprises a thin slice taken right **through** the brain. As per the earlier analogy of pulling a slice of bread out of the middle of a loaf; here a thin cross-section of the middle of the head is being isolated, showing the oval shape of the skull with the brain structures in that segment visible inside. The measurements are taken just above the ears, at the same place the paediatrician or midwife puts the measuring tape around a baby's head to get the circumference. This measurement is repeated a few times to increase accuracy. The cerebellum, ventricles,

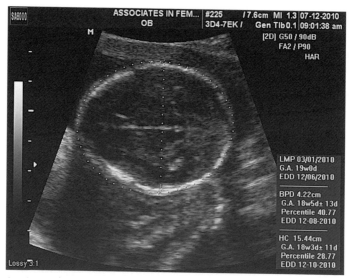

Fig. 9.1 Image showing the measurement of the BPD (biparietal diameter) and head circumference, with the corresponding gestational age. This is not the 'top' of the head, but rather a slice taken just above the level of the ears.

and other brain structures will also be evaluated and measured at different levels within the skull. By looking at these structures, multiple problems including hydrocephalus, or 'water-on-the-brain' can be ruled out.

Spine: The fetal spine will be evaluated, both in longitudinal views where it looks like a zip, and in cross-sectional views where it looks like triangular dots. In these views, open spinal defects (spina bifida) can be ruled out.

Internal organs: Careful observations are made of the fetal bladder, stomach, and kidneys, looking for blockages or obstructions. It is important to ascertain that the organs are located in their proper places, and that the diaphragm separates the heart from the stomach. The umbilical cord insertion, where it goes into the belly of the fetus, is also evaluated. The fetal abdomen should be normally closed around the cord insertion site. There should be 3 vessels identified in the umbilical cord, two arteries and one vein. A very careful evaluation of the heart and main vessels is performed; because the heart is a moving structure, this can be one of the most difficult areas to evaluate. Do not be concerned if it seems that the doctor or sonographer spends a lot of time on the heart, it often takes quite a while to acquire the right images and to confirm that everything is as it ought to be. They are checking to confirm that the four chambers in the heart are normal, and that the heart is in the proper axis within the fetal chest.

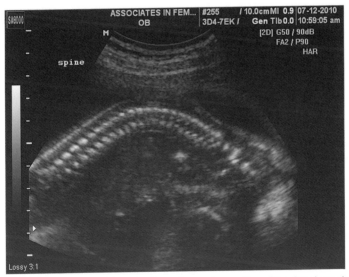

Fig. 9.2 Zipper-like view of the spine. Note the continuous line of the skin above the vertebrae (white dots) showing that it is closed. Parents often ask if it is normal that the spine appears so curved - it is!

The outflow tracts of the main vessels in the heart are also evaluated, to ensure that the vessels arise from the expected places. Often, flashes of colour can be seen if the sonographer utilizes spectral Doppler ultrasound. When the colour Doppler is turned on, you can see red and blue pulsations, which represent blood flow. This technique might be used to better evaluate the blood flow within the heart and some of the main vessels, including the umbilical cord.

Sometimes, if the images of the heart are not ideal or look suspicious, you may be referred for a fetal echocardiography. This is an ultrasound scan targeted only at the fetal heart, performed by a fetal cardiac specialist. You may also be referred for a fetal echocardiography if you have a family history or prior baby with a congenital heart defect, or if you have a medical condition or take medications that might increase the risk of a heart problem in the fetus.

Face and limbs: The fetal face is examined, with special attention paid to the lips. A cleft lip can be visualized or ruled out by taking an image that looks like the fetus is 'kissing' the screen, giving a beautiful view of the upper lip and nostrils. 3D ultrasound imaging (see Chapter 6) can also be very useful to look at the fetal face. If a defect is seen, 3D surface rendering can help the doctor and parents visualize exactly what baby looks like, and help them prepare for what they can expect at birth. 3D ultrasound also can help the physicians determine the extent of the cleft, and whether it is restricted to the lip or extends into the palate.

In the extremities, the bones should be counted, with two bones each in the lower legs and arms. The long bones are measured to ensure that they are the appropriate size. Images are taken of each foot to rule out malformed feet or a severe club foot. An attempt is made to look at the hands and fingers, but since the fists are usually closed, a totally accurate examination of each finger and toe can be limited. 3D imaging can sometimes be helpful, but rarely can both hands and feet be perfectly visualized on 2D or 3D.

Uterine environment and maternal cervix: In addition to focusing on the anatomy of the baby, a general look will be taken at the amniotic fluid volume and the uterus. They will also look at the mother's cervix, searching for signs of shortening or dilating, which can signal a preterm birth. The location of the placenta is also evaluated and documented. The placenta can be located anywhere in the uterus; a problem only arises if it is found to be blocking the cervix where the baby needs to eventually exit. If any of the placenta is seen to be very close to or covering the cervix, it is called a low-lying placenta or a placenta praevia, and it will need to be monitored very closely with follow-up ultrasounds. If it is still low after 36 weeks, a caesarean section would need to be performed. Fortunately, as the uterus grows like an expanding balloon, the placenta migrates with the uterine wall away from the cervix, and by the third trimester it is usually no longer a concern. If you are told you have a low-lying placenta, the odds of being able to deliver vaginally are still in your favour. Low-lying placentas are not uncommon in the second trimester, but only 1 in 200 or 0.5% of pregnancies have a true placenta praevia at the time of birth.

While the fundamental priority of the 20-week scan is to evaluate the fetal anatomy comprehensively, some time will often be spent on obtaining take-home photos for the parents.

If the mother is carrying twins or multiple gestations, the entire fetal survey will be repeated for each fetus. In both a singleton or multiple pregnancy, all of the required anatomy is not always well visualized, most often because the baby or babies are not in a cooperative position. In those cases, the woman may be asked to return for a follow-up scan so that the missing views can be taken.

FAQ: 'If my ultrasound scan is normal, does that mean my baby is healthy?' Verifying that the anatomy is all there and appears normal is very reassuring, but it is not a guarantee that the baby will be completely healthy at birth. Most of the time, ultrasound is reliable in ruling out physical abnormalities, but there are subtle defects that can be missed, especially in the heart. Even if the anatomy is perfect, most diseases occur in perfectly normal-looking babies. Problems with the baby's metabolism or organ function may not be detectable, nor are other non-visible problems with development such as autism.

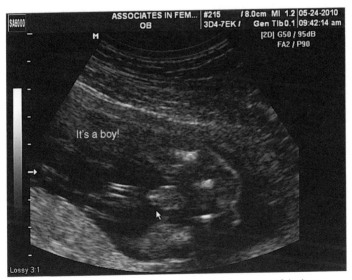

Fig. 9.3 Image of penis and scrotum between the upper portions of the legs.

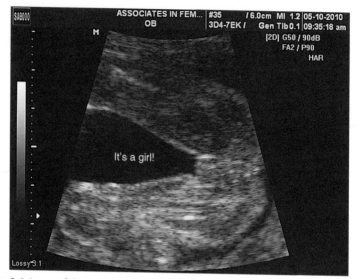

Fig. 9.4 Image of the lines or bumps of the labia between the legs.

FAQ: 'How can we tell if the baby is a boy or a girl?' In order to tell the sex, you need to see a clear shot of the anatomy, male or female. If you don't see anything, don't assume it's a girl! It means you are not looking in the right place. The best approach to see genitalia is to look at the upper thighs and rump from the bottom up. Imagine if the baby were sitting on a glass stool and you were looking up from underneath. See Figs 9.3 and 9.4.

As you can see, if the fetus insists on keeping the legs tightly together, or if it is situated so that the rump is pressed against the uterine wall, the sex can be impossible to determine. Like everything else, patience usually yields cooperation, but there are those few instances when you just cannot get a definitive answer.

FAQ: 'If they tell us it's a boy or a girl, can we be 100% sure?' If there is a good view of the gender at 20 weeks, any sonographer or doctor with experience is not going to get it wrong. One can never be 100% sure about anything, but it is highly unlikely that there would be a mistake. Sometimes patients will get additional scans later in the pregnancy, at which time the sex can be confirmed, which should erase any uncertainty. Unfortunately, there are always the rare but real case scenarios where the baby could have ambiguous genitalia, making it hard to determine the true sex even after the birth. So, while one can't predict with 100% accuracy what it will be, mistakes are rarely made with the technology available today.

FAQ: 'Is it true that you can't always tell the gender at a scan?'
Sometimes the fetus is in the wrong position, insists on keeping the legs closed, or simply isn't cooperating. If the mother is obese, that can also make it difficult to see anything, including the sex, with great detail.

FAQ: 'What if we don't want to know what sex it is?' Your doctor or sonographer will not give you this information unless you specifically request it. In some countries or centres, there may be a policy of not informing parents of the sex of the fetus. People often worry that they shouldn't even watch the scan because they are afraid they might see something to give it away. Determining the sex with confidence takes some effort, even for those who know what to look for. In the third trimester, the genitalia are much more well-formed and easy to identify, but if a woman makes it clear that she does not want to know, competent sonographers can usually complete a full scan without revealing it, and will instruct parents to look away when they may be in the relevant area. In most cases, determining and documenting the sex is not part of the ultrasound examination, nor does that information go into the woman's medical records unless an abnormality is found that might be specific to one gender versus the other, as in the case of some bladder or kidney defects. There are many myths and assumptions surrounding the sex of the fetus. Some parents may assume that because they themselves did not see male genitalia, it must be a girl. Conversely, the umbilical cord is frequently mistaken for male genitalia by parents looking at the screen. Parents have also read 'Female' on the patient records or images (this refers to the gender of the mother), and assumed it to be the sex of the child. Some people will say that because it looks active, it must be a boy, or that because the legs are crossed, it must be a girl, and so on. Be assured, there is absolutely no detectable difference in the appearance of female versus male behaviour in the womb, or the general anatomy, excluding the genitalia. Not even the heart rate (supposedly greater than 140 bpm means a girl, less than 140 bpm for a boy) is a reliable predictor, although this belief is held fast by many people.

FAQ: 'What if I don't want to know what it is, but my husband does (or vice versa)?' While the pregnancy would not have happened without his contribution, the fact remains that it is the woman who is the patient, not the man. As such, practitioners are legally bound to respect patient/physician privacy rules, and if the mother does not give permission to divulge the sex, it absolutely cannot be done, not even to the father. Of course, if the mother gives her express permission, most practices are happy to tell dad or grandma after the mother leaves the room, or write the sex on a piece of paper—whatever she permits. Despite threats from fathers, grandparents, etc, practitioners will defend the mother's right to have the ultimate say in the decision. Occasionally, fathers may insist that the mother is **not** told what sex the baby is, and while medical staff will not say anything in front of him, they will do whatever the mother requests.

FAQ: 'Do most people find out what it is?' There have not been any concrete studies on this so legitimate percentages can't be quoted, but in our experience we would say that it is about 70/30, with the majority wanting to know. It is a little more evenly divided with first pregnancies, but the scale tilts with subsequent pregnancies. After the first baby, many parents find practical reasons to want to find out what it is, such as who might have to share a room, whether they should wash the pink or blue clothes that they have been storing, should they start shopping for new things, and so forth. As mentioned previously, there may be some instances where prenatal determination of gender is not part of health policy.

Transvaginal scanning in the second trimester

The anatomy scan is almost always done by scanning abdominally. A transvaginal ultrasound would usually only be necessary in the second trimester if a patient is at felt to be at risk for preterm birth. Risk factors for preterm labour include multiple miscarriages or pregnancy terminations, carrying twins (or more), prior pre-term birth, or a history of biopsy or surgery on the cervix. In these cases, your provider may opt to perform a series of transvaginal measurements of the cervix between approximately 16 and 24 weeks to ensure that the cervix is showing no signs of shortening or dilating. Should the cervix demonstrate troubling signs of prematurely opening, there are some preventative strategies that your provider may opt to employ depending on your situation and history.

Soft markers

Soft markers have been the cause of a lot of anxiety over the years as ultrasound screening has evolved. Countless families have been alarmed to hear that their fetus has a soft marker, when in fact it turned out that they were having a perfectly normal baby. 'Soft markers' is a term for certain anatomical variations that are neither abnormal nor cause problems in the fetus, but have been loosely correlated as a possible flag for Down's syndrome. Soft markers are minor, subtle findings in the fetal anatomy that tend to resolve spontaneously, and almost always have no clinically significant consequences to the health or development of the baby. There are six main ones that can be found at the anatomy scan:

- Thickness to the skin folds at the back of the neck (slightly different from nuchal translucency which is a collection of fluid under the skin at 11–13 weeks)

- Small collection of fluid in the collecting system of the kidneys, known as pyelectasis

- Echogenic (bright) areas within the bowel

- Choroid plexus cysts in the brain

- Echogenic (bright) spot in a chamber of the heart

- Shorter than expected long bones of the arms or legs

While these anatomical differences sound scary or serious, they are rarely abnormal. With advancements in the ability to see very fine detail within the fetus, most of these are things that had never been observed before, and the medical community simply didn't know what they meant. Over time, after gathering data on many thousands of babies, countless studies have shown that these are almost always benign, inconsequential findings that don't even require follow up. They are just normal isolated variations in fetal development. However, as doctors and researchers were dedicating their time and practice to trying to find any possible signal that the fetus might have a genetic abnormality, a lot has been made of these findings. In the process, it was found that there was indeed a statistical link between these markers and babies found to have Down's syndrome or Trisomy 13 or 18. So, it became the standard of practice to take note of these soft markers and discuss with parents that if any of these are present, it increased the risk of their baby being abnormal and invasive testing might be considered.

In the last decade, the trend has been that the discovery of a single soft marker in an otherwise low-risk fetus should not be taken in isolation and interpreted as something that significantly increases risk. A single soft marker usually does not increase the risk of having an abnormal baby enough to be of any concern. However, soft markers would be considered a red flag if there were more than one, if they occurred in the context of other anatomical abnormalities, or if they were detected in conjunction with a marginal/abnormal screening blood test, or advanced maternal age. Some markers, such as fluid in the kidneys or a bright spot in the heart, do very little to statistically increase your risk, while significantly shortened thigh bones or a very thick neck carry more weight. Doctors have developed statistical methods to calculate how to integrate soft markers with other findings, in order to revise risk calculations and help women and their partners decide whether further testing is appropriate.

The bottom line is that if you are told that one of these soft markers has been found at your scan, do not panic. It does not mean your baby has a birth defect or has Down's syndrome. Most of the time is doesn't mean anything at all except to put doctors in the awkward position of trying to explain them to parents without causing undue alarm.

10

Third trimester ultrasound and NST

➜ Key points

- Third trimester scans are not always routinely performed.

- The primary medical reasons to have an ultrasound are to check the growth of the fetus, assess the amniotic fluid volume, check the position (breech versus head-first), or to look for signs of fetal distress.

- Valuable medical information can be gained at the later stages of the pregnancy with ultrasound, but good take-home photos are not always possible.

- A biophysical profile is a type of ultrasound scan that assesses the well-being of the fetus. It is sometimes performed in conjunction with a non-stress test (NST).

A third trimester scan is not always necessary in every pregnancy. Once the anatomic scan at 18–20 weeks has demonstrated a normal-appearing fetus with all of the appropriate body parts, there is usually no need to reassess the anatomy as it is not likely to change. However, in the general routine testing of the mother (see Chapter 2) and for various other reasons, sometimes your provider will want to take another look with the ultrasound. Some practices might recommend a routine third trimester ultrasound, depending on where you live and the accepted standard of care. However, if things are progressing normally, a scan in the third trimester might not be warranted financially without a compelling medical reason.

Medical indications for a scan

One of the most common reasons for an ultrasound scan in the third trimester is to get a good indication of fetal growth and to monitor the amniotic fluid volume. Things that might affect growth and fluid are maternal type I, II, or gestational diabetes, high blood pressure, or a prior history of having an unusually large or small baby. Sometimes, even in the absence of those other risk factors, the provider may feel that the uterus is smaller or larger than expected and will want to use ultrasound to investigate.

The doctor or midwife can usually determine the fetal position with confidence by feeling the mother's belly with their hands. By 36 weeks, the fetus is expected to have assumed the head-down position (also known as vertex or cephalic presentation) where it will remain until birth. If the provider suspects that the fetus is not head-down, or is unsure as to where the head really is, they might order an ultrasound to confirm the position. Towards the very end of the pregnancy, if the head is not vertex, ultrasound can be used to guide the doctors should they decide to try to manually turn the baby around in preparation for a vaginal birth. This manoeuvre is known as an external cranial version, and would almost always be done under direct ultrasound guidance.

If the location of the placenta had been a concern earlier on, your provider will order an ultrasound to see whether the cervix is clear. If special attention needs to be paid to the cervix, the scan might be performed transvaginally, but otherwise the evaluation of the fetus in the third trimester will be done transabdominally. Late in the pregnancy, a targeted ultrasound can be performed to assess fetal well being, known as a **biophysical profile**. This is most likely to be done if the pregnancy goes beyond the due date.

What can be seen in the third trimester on an ultrasound scan?

Often, not too much! At least, you may not be able to see much in the way of a recognizable baby. Parents are sometimes disappointed at how little they can see after 28 weeks, expecting that since the baby is so much bigger and developed, it should be easier to see. Unfortunately, the opposite is often true. By now, the fetal bones have begun to harden and calcify. Ultrasound cannot see through hard bone so the arms, legs, and spine cast shadows everywhere. In addition, the body parts are so big that the head alone takes up the whole monitor, compared to the anatomy scan when the entire baby could fit into that same space. The fetal face is usually wedged down into the mother's lower pelvis, which is great in preparation for the birth, but not so great for getting a picture.

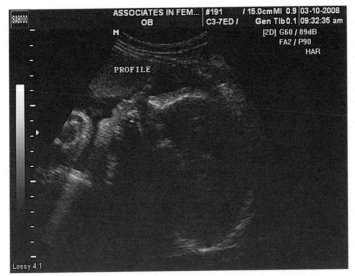

Fig. 10.1 32 week fetal profile in a baby facing up. Notice the head takes up most of the screen, and the heavy shadowing caused by the jaw, skull, and arm bones.

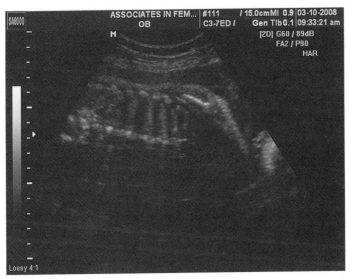

Fig. 10.2 Rib and spine shadows in a 32 week fetus.

Fetal size

It may be hard to get photos for the baby album, but some valuable diagnostic information can be gained from a late ultrasound scan. Measurements of the fetal head, abdomen, and femur bones are taken. Tables within the ultrasound machine use that information to calculate an estimate of fetal weight. It is important to emphasize that fetal weights given by ultrasound are an **estimation**, not an exact prediction. You can imagine that weighing yourself by taking the length of your thigh, the circumference of your belly, and the circumference of your head and plugging that into a mathematical formula is not likely to give you your true weight. The accepted range is plus or minus 10%, approximately 350 grams or 0.75 lbs, towards the end of the pregnancy. While this may sound very inexact, it can be a valuable guide to your provider when fetal size is suspiciously small or large.

FAQ: 'The ultrasound says my baby is 2 weeks ahead in size. Does this mean my due date changes?' Usually, your due date is well established by the end of the first trimester. It is not appropriate to adjust a due date in the third trimester based on the size of the baby. It is important to reiterate that a 'due date' is only the date that marks the 40th week of the pregnancy, not necessarily the day you are expected to give birth. With each measurement the sonographer takes, the machine calculates an average gestational age. For example, if the thigh bone measures 7.2 cm, this corresponds to a gestational age of 36 weeks and 4 days. That same baby may have an abdominal circumference of 31.3 cm. which corresponds to a gestational age of 35 weeks and 1 day. All of the many measurements that are taken will each come up with a different corresponding age. It is expected that each measurement will be off by a few days or even a couple of weeks. This is normal as long as they fall within the expected general range. The machine averages all the measurements together to come up with a final estimate of gestational age based on size alone. This is then compared against the known, established gestational age of the fetus in order to get an idea of whether the baby is growing at the 25th or the 75th percentile or whatever it may be. If you come out 2 weeks ahead in size, then your baby has not advanced in time, but is instead bigger than average. Your provider may make decisions about when you should give birth based on the size, but that's not the same as changing a due date.

The amniotic fluid index

In the third trimester, amniotic fluid volume is assessed by taking a measurement of the deepest pockets of fluid in each of the four quadrants of the uterus. These measurements are added together to come up with a single number known as the AFI, or amniotic fluid index. The threshold for concern may vary from practice to practice, but in general, if the AFI is below 7 or 8, the fluid is considered abnormally low. This condition is known as oligohydram-nios. There are many reasons why the fluid volume may be inadequate, but regardless of the cause, a low fluid level is an indicator that the uterine envi-ronment may no longer be optimal. Conversely, if there is too much fluid, known as polyhydramnios, that can be a concern as well.

Biophysical profile

Late in the pregnancy, if there are concerns about fluid, decreased fetal move-ments, or if you go beyond your due date, your doctor might recommend a biophysical profile ultrasound. This is a specific, targeted scan performed to assess fetal well being. In addition to calculating an amniotic fluid index, the sonographer and/or doctor will be looking for fetal movements such as kick-ing, rolling, flexing of the body, and the sucking reflex. They will also look for sustained fetal 'breathing'. Obviously, the fetus is not breathing air yet, but if you watch the chest area, you can actually see the diaphragm moving up and down, and the abdomen and ribs contracting and expanding. Seeing these movements is reassuring because it indicates that the fetus is receiving ade-quate oxygen at the deepest parts of its brain, and is able to expend energy moving, exercising, and building the muscle tone it will need to breathe and function well outside of the womb. If there is a good amniotic fluid index, good fetal movements, and prolonged breathing movements for 30 seconds or so, the fetus gets a passing score for the biophysical test.

Often, a biophysical profile will be done in conjunction with a non-stress test (NST). An NST is another method to assess the overall well-being of the fetus. It is done by attaching one or two flat, round disc-like monitors to the mother's abdomen which is held securely by an elastic belt. The mother sits quietly in a reclining chair or examination bed while the monitor runs for at least 20 minutes to a half hour. The monitor is simultaneously recording a tracing of the fetal heart beat and any uterine contractions that may be occur-ring. The mother is also given a button to press every time she feels the baby moving or kicking. The test is considered reactive (good) if the baby's heart rate accelerates as it should in response to movement or contractions, at least twice in a 20 minute period. If, after 20 minutes, the baby hasn't moved much or there haven't been sufficient uterine contractions, they might try giving the mother a glass of juice or something sugary to get the baby moving. If they suspect the baby is just taking a nice deep nap, sometimes they will try to wake it up by pressing a buzzer onto the mother's abdomen which is painless for both the mother and fetus, but often provokes some action.

FAQ: 'Can we tell by ultrasound if the baby's lungs are developed?' No. Ultrasound can see that the lungs are there and appear normal, but whether or not the lungs are mature enough to adequately oxygenate the blood after the baby is born is something that can simply not be seen. Sometimes, while watching the fetus, the chest will expand and contract and it will look just like it is breathing. These fetal respirations are reassuring that the fetus is not in distress but they are <u>not</u> a sign that the lungs are ready. These instinctive reflexes can be seen in fetuses as early as 16 to 20 weeks gestation. If an early birth (before 37–38 weeks) is likely to be needed, doctors can use ultrasound to guide an amniocentesis, or sampling of amniotic fluid, which can be chemically analyzed to definitively determine if the lungs are mature.

'What is fetal scalp monitoring?' Once your labour is underway, you may spend some time hooked up to a cardiotocograph to monitor your contractions and your baby's heart rate. This is the same machine that they use for the non-stress test (NST) where a large elastic band with one or two small disc-like monitors is placed around your abdomen. This will help your midwife or obstetrician assess how frequent and strong your contractions are, and how well the fetus is responding to the stresses of labour. Your midwife or obstetrician may feel that they want a more accurate means of monitoring the baby and may opt to use a fetal scalp electrode. This is a thin metal wire that is placed just under the skin on the fetal scalp and is a reliable method to observe any changes in the fetal heart rate that might signal fetal distress while you labor. This is not necessarily used routinely in normal labours unless clinically indicated.

11

Options if an abnormality is found

➔ Key points

- Fortunately, severe abnormalities are relatively uncommon, affecting only about 3% of pregnancies. However, the types of abnormalities that can occur are numerous and need to be addressed on an individual basis with your providers and specialists.

- Counselling and support are very important if your pregnancy is found to be abnormal. Support groups can be an invaluable source of information and help.

- Referral to a maternal fetal medicine specialist and additional testing will almost always be necessary to confirm the diagnosis, discuss prognosis, and learn about potential interventions.

- Visits to additional specialists who are experts in the field of your specific anomaly can also be helpful.

- Once an abnormality is confirmed, a decision needs to be made by the parents as to whether interventions are desired or whether pregnancy termination is an option.

- Pregnancy terminations are subject to limitations depending on gestational age and local laws.

Fortunately, major abnormalities in pregnancies that have not spontaneously miscarried before 8 or 9 weeks are uncommon. Should you find yourself among those who have received bad news about your pregnancy, you will be struggling with a multitude of emotions; shock, fear, sadness, grief, sometimes even anger or guilt. The most important thing will be to seek out support systems that can help you move forward. You may want to turn to trusted family, friends, or clergy for advice, and you may find it helpful to seek professional help or counselling. This can be a very stressful period, made more difficult by the fact that there is often only a small window of time to make a decision about whether or not you want to continue with the pregnancy, if that is an option for you. The timing of termination is subject to legal limits, with 22 to 24 weeks being the latest in most places. Under special circumstances, it is possible to obtain a later termination, but not all providers have the necessary skill and you may have to travel. In order to make a decision regarding termination, or to prepare for life after the birth, you will need to learn as much as possible about the diagnosis and the prognosis. Many families obtain second opinions from specialists with expertise in the specific abnormality.

Again, the number of pregnancies that are actually afflicted with a severe abnormality (also known as anomaly) are very small, roughly 3%. However, the variety of abnormalities that can occur is huge, far too many to be adequately addressed in a single book such as this. Your providers will be able to address your specific needs and best explain your individual options. The following is a guide to the general process regarding the interventions and resources that may be available to you should you receive bad news. We have also included a list of websites in the appendix that you may find helpful.

Anatomical abnormalities

There is an obvious distinction between some severe abnormalities versus minor abnormalities. For example, blindness is severe as opposed to the more minor case of poor vision corrected with glasses. Unfortunately, in the realm of prenatal testing, this distinction isn't always clear, even with the most advanced technologies available today. If an abnormality is found, it may be hard for the doctors to tell how significant a problem it might be. It can be very frustrating to be told that they think the baby has abnormality, but they don't know the severity of it, if it will require treatment or surgery, or how negatively it may impact the baby after it is born. Often, they truly cannot predict how the anomaly might progress. Some defects such as blockages or some tumors can spontaneously regress or even resolve. In other instances, they steadily progress to the point of permanent organ damage or even fetal or neonatal death. It is very important to get as much expert information as you can, but also to communicate your needs and beliefs to your providers so that they can most effectively guide you through your options.

Genetic testing

In many cases, if a defect is suspected, your provider is likely to offer you genetic testing, even if your screening tests showed no increased risk. Many physical abnormalities, even minor ones, can be a symptom of a larger genetic or chromosomal problem. Information obtained from the fetal chromosomes would be tremendously helpful in determining the prognosis and extent of the potential impairments. In addition, certain chromosomal abnormalities have a very poor prognosis for survival; many don't even make it to term. Knowing that the fetus is chromosomally abnormal might help you in your decision to either let nature take its course, to terminate, or to refuse medical interventions such as surgery or resuscitation after birth. If you decide to continue with the pregnancy, you can work towards being prepared for all possible eventualities. In the case of Down's syndrome or others where death is much less likely, you can make preparations to learn about the disorder and meet the needs and challenges that will lie ahead.

Further testing/second opinions

If you have been told your baby has a problem, the chances are you will make quite a few visits to various professionals before you have a complete understanding of your situation. If you have not already visited a high-risk maternal fetal medicine centre to consult with perinatologists, this will probably be your next step. They have excellent imaging capabilities and are able to expertly advise you about the specific abnormality that your fetus has, and the potential interventions that may be available.

They will also be able to point you in the direction of other specialists who would need to be involved with the treatment of the child once it is born. For example, if a cleft lip (harelip) is found, the perinatologists can determine the general extent of the defect, whether it is confined to just the lip, or extends deep into the palate, etc. This information can then be taken to a maxillofacial surgeon who is experienced in repairing these problems in infancy and childhood. You can meet with the surgeons and staff before your baby is born so everything can be explained. Meanwhile, you may want to start doing some research yourself as well. If you have not already been directed to a support group by the involved physicians or their staff, finding and joining a support group of people who have endured similar challenges can be tremendously helpful and educational. Discovering that your baby has a cleft lip is definitely upsetting, but if the baby is otherwise normal, learning about how to overcome the initial feeding difficulties and the brilliant repairs that can be done usually helps parents accept the challenge and cope well. Unfortunately, not all anomalies have such a bright outlook. However, knowing more about them will help you formulate a plan of management.

Fetal MRI

In cases where additional information can affect decision-making about continuing a pregnancy or planning for care after birth, a fetal MRI might be done.

MRI stands for Magnetic Resonance Imaging and is considered safe for newborns, children, and adults. It is probably quite safe to use in pregnancy, but this is still under investigation. However, in these cases its use is well justified. It can be technically difficult to get good MRI images as the pictures are affected by the motion of the fetus. Even so, valuable information about the exact nature and extent of the fetal abnormality can be gained.

Genetic counselling

Many maternal fetal medicine centres work very closely with genetic counsellors, who may be part of your counselling process. Genetic counsellors take detailed family and medical histories and can assess the chances of disease occurrence or recurrence. They can help the medical team in advising you, if your pregnancy is affected by a chromosomal or gene defect. Even if you do not consult with a genetic counsellor during this difficult time, you may wish to talk to one before your next pregnancy. They can help reassure you or advise you as to the likelihood of subsequent pregnancies being similarly affected.

Making a decision

Once you've learned about the defects, prognosis, and potential interventions as thoroughly as you can, you and your partner can make an informed decision about how to proceed. Again, we stress the importance of finding a support group for families who are dealing with issues similar to yours. Many large hospitals with speciality children's centres will have support groups, or information on how to find one. There are also many of these groups on the internet, where you can read blogs, post concerns, and get some good advice. Even so, remember that in the end, the decision is still **yours** to make. Everybody you talk to may have an opinion, but you and your partner are going to be the ones who have the ultimate responsibility for the care of the baby once it is born. There are so many factors to consider: the medical details, your personal circumstances, the emotional and economic burden, and so forth. It's not possible to please everyone, so do your best to find what is right for you.

Medical interventions

If you choose to continue the pregnancy, you will still have some decisions to make. Your providers may refer you to specialists, or you may prefer to do some research and find your own specialists. Some cutting-edge treatments, and certain types of fetal and neonatal surgeries, may only be available at a few places in each country, and some treatments are still experimental. It may be necessary for you to temporarily relocate to one of these centres, where you will eventually give birth and where the baby will be cared for as a newborn, sometimes for months. If the prognosis for your pregnancy is grave, you always have the option of letting nature take its course. You have the right to balance the prognosis for survival against the economic and emotional costs of intervening. Some mothers prefer to give birth closer to home and request palliative, comfort-based care for the newborn, rather than opting for surgery or other procedures that have only a small chance of success.

If you are in a position where you want to try anything and everything possible, fetal surgery can sometimes be performed by making an incision in the uterus to allow access to the fetus. This is usually only performed in cases where survival after birth is unlikely without some intervention. There is a significant risk of adverse outcomes, due to infection or premature labour, so this route is usually reserved for drastic cases. Less invasive and less risky interventions can sometimes be performed using microsurgical techniques. In certain cases this can be done very successfully. Good results are regularly obtained by the placement of shunts (tubes) in cases where fluid is accumulating in the fetus, which can improve the success of further surgical procedures after delivery. The high-risk centres can also offer the latest in medical therapies, fetal blood transfusions, and special delivery techniques for babies whose breathing may be compromised. Again, there is such a wide range of possible anomalies and treatments, it is impossible to address them all here. The key point is that if you know in advance that your baby is going to have certain problems, you can arrange to give birth at a facility that is best equipped for your specific needs, with a team prepared to deliver the most appropriate care.

Pregnancy terminations

Having been told that their fetus has a serious anatomical and/or chromosomal defect, many women will choose to end the pregnancy. Chemical pregnancy terminations, which use medication that causes miscarriage, can be performed before 8 weeks. However, since it is virtually impossible to determine whether abnormalities exist prior to 8 weeks gestation with current technology, a surgical termination is the more likely option. Surgical termination may also be required if the fetus has died in the womb for any reason. Your provider will advise you on your best options, which will be affected by the duration of the pregnancy and the specific methods available in your area or country. There are three basic procedures used for a termination of pregnancy (also known as TOP), D&C, D&E, and induction of labour, which are explained in detail below. Some bleeding and cramping can be expected for a few days after any of these procedures. It is very important to return for a follow-up visit after the procedure, so that the provider can ensure that there is no retained material and check for signs of infection.

D&C (Dilatation and curettage)

This type of procedure can only be done up until 12–14 weeks. Under local or (more typically) general anaesthesia, the cervix is gradually opened by inserting thin metal dilators. A suction device is inserted and the contents of the uterus are removed. This procedure has the lowest complication rates, and is preferable to terminating pregnancies later in gestation. Unfortunately, it can often be difficult to obtain a diagnosis and make a decision in time for this procedure to be performed.

D&E (Dilatation and evacuation)

This type of procedure is usually performed after 13 weeks. It is similar to a D&C, except that instead of using a vacuum cannula (suction tube), the uterine contents are extracted with specialized instruments. This procedure is slightly riskier than first trimester D&C, but the risk of complications is generally low in the hands of qualified and experienced personnel.

Induction of labour

In the second and third trimesters of pregnancy, induction of labour is sometimes necessary as the method used to end the pregnancy. Third trimester terminations are usually performed only in cases of severe and lethal fetal abnormalities; clinical practice will depend on local and national regulations. Labour may also be induced in the third trimester following spontaneous fetal death in the womb. Usually, the cervix is first primed with hormones to enable dilation. Labour is started by rupturing the amniotic sac and by administering intravenous medications. In many places, the fetus will be given a lethal injection under ultrasound guidance up to three days prior to an induction of labor or a D&E, which can lower the risk of complications. Whether or not a D&E or induction of labour is attempted is often dependent upon the preferences and skills of the participating doctors.

12

More frequently asked questions

'I think I may be leaking amniotic fluid. What type of test can be done to check?' Your provider can do a nitrazine test and/or a fern test to check whether or not amniotic fluid may be leaking from the vagina. For the nitrazine test, a swab of the vaginal fluid is taken and the pH is tested using a strip of nitrazine paper. Amniotic fluid has a higher pH than normal vaginal secretions, so if the strip shows the pH to be elevated, you are probably leaking fluid. A fern test may also be performed, where a swab of vaginal fluid is taken and placed on a slide where it is allowed to air-dry. Your provider can look at the dried fluid on the slide to see if there is the presence of fern-like patterns of crystals. If fern-like crystals are seen, you are leaking amniotic fluid. These tests are about 85-100% accurate; however, they can be misleading if there is bleeding or an active vaginal infection.

There are also over-the-counter tests that you can buy to use at home. They are basically panty liners with an indicator strip. A change of color means a positive result, in which case you should call your provider. These can also be misleading in the presence of a vaginal infection. Even if your home test is negative, if you feel that you have been leaking fluid and you are at all concerned, contact your provider for an evaluation.

'Last time they told me my baby's heart rate was 157. Today it's 142. Is something wrong?' No, differences in heart rates from moment-to-moment or day-to-day is a good thing since it shows that the fetal heart rate is *variable*. Variability demonstrates that the heart rate is responsive to the changing oxygen needs of the fetus, and is a sign of fetal well-being. If you were to run up the stairs, your heart rate would increase, and if you were sitting or napping, your heart rate would drop accordingly. The same principles apply to the fetus. A sleeping fetus is going to have a lower heart rate than one who is jumping and kicking. Variablity is reassuring, it isn't normal for a fetal heart rate to stay constant.

'How can they tell the heart rate with ultrasound?' Heart rates can be documented either with Doppler ultrasound, which allows you to hear the

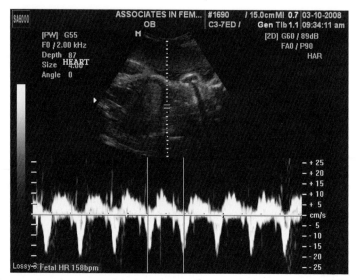

Fig. 12.1 Doppler tracing of the heart beat. The rate is calculated by measuring the distance between peaks.

heart beating, or a linear tracing of the heart motion. The Doppler feature, which gives the audible sound of the heartbeat, should not regularly be used in early pregnancy so as to minimize exposure of the embryo to excessive ultrasound energy. However, Doppler and colour Doppler (another high-tech form of Doppler) ultrasound can be used in the second and third trimester. These techniques are useful for evaluating the blood flow within the fetus, especially the fetal heart and outflow tracts. It can also be used on the umbilical cord to investigate whether there might be problems with blood flow between the placenta and the fetus. In some instances, the blood flow through the placenta and cord might become restricted or impeded, and the fetus will struggle to get enough oxygen and valuable nutrients. Serial Doppler studies can be used to monitor the pregnancy if this becomes a concern.

'What are kick counts?' Starting around 7 or 8 months, your provider may ask you to do kick counts. Kick counts are an indirect way to test the health and well being of the fetus. This is done on a daily basis, but pick the time of day when the fetus is most likely to be active. Don't choose a time when you know your baby tends to be quiet or napping, or when you will be too busy to really be aware of the fetal activity. On a piece of paper, write down the time you start, and make a mark each time you feel a movement. Once you get to 10 movements, you have finished the test. Usually, you should have noted 10 movements within two hours. If two hours have passed and you haven't gotten 10 movements, try drinking some fruit juice or having a snack and try again. If 4 hours have passed and still you have not gotten 10 movements, you should call your provider who will possibly bring you to the clinic for an assessment, and possibly do an NST (non-stress test) or ultrasound.

'I'm 5 months pregnant, and I still don't feel the baby moving much. Is something wrong?' If at any point in the pregnancy, you notice a decrease in fetal movements, or you haven't felt the baby kick in a while, you should definitely call your care provider. Most of the time, everything is fine but it is better to be cautious than to ignore it. However, around 4 and 5 months, most people are only just beginning to feel the fetus regularly, and it is too early to do effective kick counts. Some women will feel active kicking as early as 16 weeks, but others may take another month or two, making them wonder why they aren't feeling anything yet. Or, mothers will be very anxious because in prior pregnancies, they felt movements earlier and worry that this baby doesn't move as much as their last one did. In many of these cases, ultrasound will show that the placenta is located anteriorly, or on the front of the uterus (the part behind the mother's skin and belly button). The placenta can be located

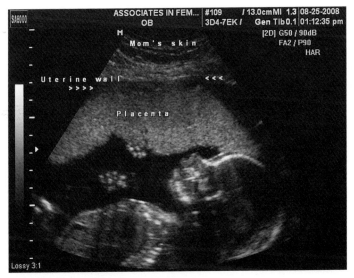

Fig. 12.2 Ultrasound image of anterior placenta.

anywhere in the uterus, its position is only of concern if it is blocking the cervix where the fetus needs to exit. An anterior placenta is harmless, but may mean that the mother **perceives** less fetal movement. The front of the uterus is the most sensitive to kicks and bumps from the fetus, but if the placenta is there, it can act as a cushion or buffer between the mother and the fetus. Often, as the pregnancy progresses and the fetus grows bigger, the movements will be felt more vigorously. However, there are some cases where women will have a difficult time feeling the movements throughout the whole pregnancy, even with a healthy, active baby. Knowing that you have an anterior placenta can explain the lack of sensitivity.

'When is the best time to get good 3D pictures?' The 12 week 3D ultrasound pictures can be interesting, but parents sometimes think the fetus looks more like a grasshopper or an alien than a baby. It's too early to see what the baby is really going to look like when he or she is born. For scans where it will really look like your baby, the best time to get 3D pictures is around 25 to 28 weeks. By this time, the fetus has put on some body fat, and the face has started to show individuality. Before this, fetuses can look very skinny and skeletal, and many parents feel that they even look frightening. After 30 weeks, the fetal head is usually wedged down in the maternal pelvis, since the fetus is starting to run out of room, and it is difficult to get an unobstructed view of the face. See Figs 12.3–12.7.

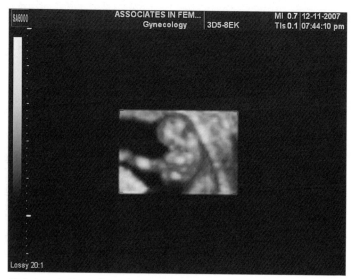

Fig. 12.3 9 week 3D – beluga whale versus human?

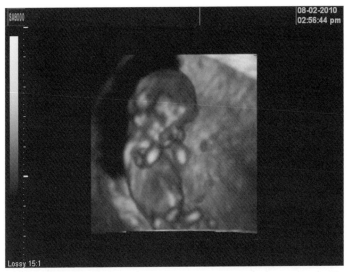

Fig. 12.4 15 week 3D – recognizably human, but no individuality yet and overall look can be unnerving.

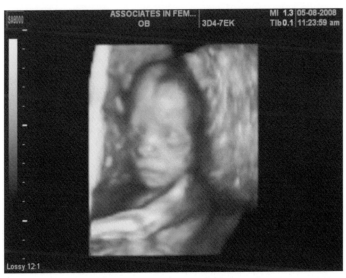

Fig. 12.5 Another 20 week 3D. This fetus is in a great position and photogenic, but the lack of body fat typical at this time in the gestation gives it a skeletal, wax-figure appearance.

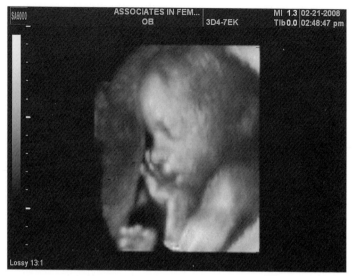

Fig. 12.6 26 week 3D – now that's a beautiful baby!

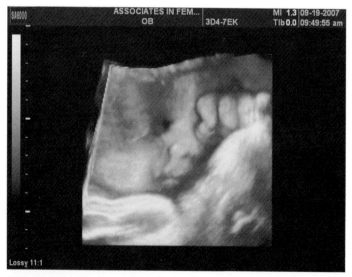

Fig. 12.7 34 weeks: Here is a small window to get a nice shot of the side of the face. However, you can see how much of the face is obstructed by the hand and upper arm. In addition, the fuzzy bit up in the left corner may look like hair, but in fact, it is part of the uterine wall.

'Can we see if the baby has hair?' You can see hair sometimes, but usually only in the third trimester, and only on 2D ultrasound. On 3D, the computer processes the surface rendered image so that sometimes it looks like there is hair, but it is only an effect of clever shading. On 2D, if the fetus has hair can be seen as little wisps floating in the fluid outside the scalp or towards the neck.

'Why can't I see the baby very well on my ultrasound?' Sometimes patients will be disappointed because the images aren't as clear as they expect. Timing, fetal cooperation, position, and the amount of amniotic fluid are crucial factors in whether or not you can get a good 3D or even 2D picture. As with any photo shoot, whether or not you get a decent picture is dependent on circumstances completely beyond medical or maternal control, such as how photogenic or cooperative the fetus is at the moment.

Even if the scanning is being done at the optimal time and the fetus is in a good position, maternal size also plays a large role in the clarity of the image. It is a basic and unavoidable law of ultrasound physics that with increasing depth or penetration comes decreased resolution. To put it more simply, the more abdominal fat there is, the further the sound beam will have to travel and the worse the image will be.

'Now that I've taken my ultrasound pictures home, I've begun to wonder if the baby really looks normal?' Getting 2D and 3D ultrasound pictures can be a lot of fun, and it is especially exciting to watch the fetus 'live' or in 4D. At the end of the scan, parents are often given some keepsake photos to take home and show family and friends. After studying the images and trying to explain to grandma what the picture represents, parents will often become confused or worried that that some vague area in their picture might actually represent something wrong that was 'missed'. It is not at all uncommon for us to get phone calls or visits from concerned women, clutching their photos and asking for us to explain why 'the hand looks funny' or 'what is that growing out of my baby's head?' It must be stressed that 3D images are not actual photographs like you would take of a person standing in front of you. Rather, they are **computer-constructed** images created from data acquired through sound pulses. In order for the ultrasound machine to generate an image, it needs to filter out a lot of extraneous noise and make a lot of assumptions. Plus, there is interference from surrounding structures such as the uterine wall, placenta, limbs, and so forth and the computer doesn't know to separate these from the fetus. These floating objects and details often aren't flattering to the overall appearance. As a result, some strange things can appear to happen. The sonographer does his/her best to maximize the image, usually focusing on the best features that can be seen, but there are almost always some drawbacks elsewhere in the picture.

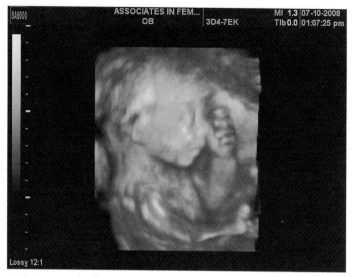

Fig. 12.8 An example of 3D's limitations. The 'brains' of the ultrasound machine are focused on this beautiful profile and left hand. However, the near side of the head, shoulder, and arm look funny. This is simply because of technical limitations, not because the baby is malformed. In this case, if visualization of the arm and shoulder were to look perfect, the profile and left hand wouldn't have looked as good.

Both 2D and 3D ultrasound can sometimes be like a Rorschach Ink Blot test; one person sees a bat while another sees a lizard. When you are in the ultrasound room watching the picture live, it's easier for your brain to assimilate the information and things don't look too strange. But once you take those still-frame pictures home and stare at them for a while, you might start to see all sorts of strange things to worry about. Rest assured, your baby is just fine!

FAQ: 'It looks like the cord is near the baby's neck. Isn't that dangerous?'
One drawback to utilizing 3D is that the umbilical cord is often clearly seen in the region of the head and neck. In fact, this happens more often than it doesn't, and it almost always invokes a lot of concern from parents. On 2D pictures, it may be there but it just isn't obvious to most parents. The umbilical cord extends outward from the fetal abdomen (at the place that eventually becomes the belly button) and is normally quite long. A lengthy, coiled cord is a good thing since it gives the fetus freedom of movement during its time in the womb, and allows for unrestrained descent of the fetus through the birth canal at birth. All too often, we can see the cord actually wrapping around the neck. This is probably one of the biggest downsides to 3D and 4D scanning, since it can be very hard to reassure parents that this is not abnormal, dangerous,

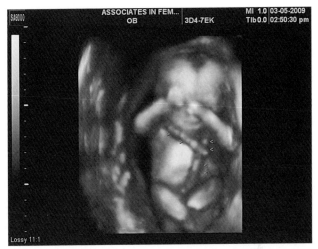

Fig. 12.9 This 16 week fetus can be seen with the cord wrapped around it like a necktie. Certainly this is looks alarming, but it rarely causes a problem. By the 20 week anatomy scan, this fetus was completely necktie-free.

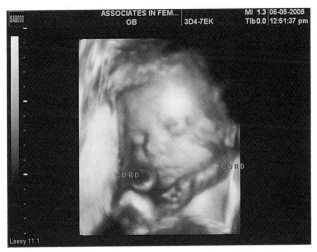

Fig. 12.10 This image was used in a US clinic as a promotional picture. Providers are so used to seeing the cord at the neck that little attention was paid to its presence. However, instead of commenting on the beautiful face, this image has prompted hundreds of questions from concerned patients that this fetus could be 'in danger'. It therefore ended up being used mostly as a talking point about the normal appearance of the cord at the neck. This baby was born vaginally without incident.

or cause for alarm. The fact is that the cord will be around the neck in approximately **25%** of all pregnancies. Fortunately, babies being strangled to death in the womb is exceedingly rare, less than 1%. So, in the very likely event that the cord is seen in the region of the fetal head or around the neck, do not expect that you are high risk or that your doctor is going to do anything about it. It is **not** a reason to do follow up scans, initiate an early birth, or do an elective caesarean.

'**How does ultrasound calculate the age of the baby?**' A few groups of researchers painstakingly collected data at various points in fetal development and created tables with normal parameters of biometrics (body part measurements). Almost every body part and organ has a table with corresponding ranges of sizes to age. These tables have been embedded into the ultrasound software so that when a specific body part is measured, a corresponding age/date is calculated. The most important measurement in the first trimester is the crown-rump length which is a measurement of the embryo from end to end. In the 2nd and 3rd trimesters, the head circumference, skull diameter, abdominal circumference, humerus (arm), and femur (leg) bones are the typical standards against which the growth of the fetus is judged. Rarely do all these body parts all measure exactly to the day what they are supposed to according to the known age of the fetus. Each body part has an acceptable range, which has been compiled and built into the tables. As long as the measurements are within that range, growth is considered normal.

'**Is there a test that can tell me how much the baby will weigh at birth?**' A truly accurate and dependable prediction of birth weight would be a valuable test indeed! As many people will attest, despite all the technology there can be a great discrepancy between predicted birth weight and the true weight. One way your provider tracks the growth of the fetus is to measure the size of the uterus, done by measuring the distance from the pubic bone to the top of the uterus, known as the fundus. This is a very simple yet elegant way to measure growth, as each centimeter is equivalent to approximately 1 week of gestation. By 20 weeks, the fundus should lie 20 cm from the pubic bone (this happens to be roughly the position of the navel); at 30 weeks it should lie 30 cm from the pubic bone, etc. However, this obviously isn't foolproof as many factors can affect the measurement such as whether the mother is short or long-waisted, if the fetus is lying in an unusual position, or if there is a large amount of maternal belly fat making it hard to feel the top of the uterus. Amniotic fluid is also an invisible factor that the provider cannot detect simply by measuring fundal height. Under normal circumstances, there can be a large variance in the amount of amniotic fluid surrounding the fetus. A large amount of fluid is going to take up space within the uterus, increasing the fundal height and making it seem like there is a much bigger fetus inside. If the provider feels that the uterine size is greater or smaller than the dates, an ultrasound may be ordered in an attempt to get a more accurate assessment of what might be going on in the uterus.

With ultrasound, fetal weights are calculated by applying a mathematical equation to the size of the fetal head and abdomen. In order for the algorithm to provide a reliable estimated weight, precise measurements of the head and abdomen need to be obtained. Unfortunately, towards the end of the pregnancy, the fetal head is usually wedged deep into the mother's pelvis, making an accurate measurement difficult. To further compound the potential for inaccuracy, the fetal body is also tightly curled and bent with the knees and arms pressing against the belly, limiting the likelihood of getting a true and accurate measurement around the abdomen. Since these are the two crucial measurements required to get an estimated weight, very often the weight predicted is not as reliable as one would like, with a plus or minus range of approximately 10% or 0.75 lb. Estimated fetal weights really are **estimates**, not predictions.

'The doctor says my due date is Jan. 10, but at my 20 week scan the ultrasound says I'm due Jan. 15. Which do I believe?' The only time the ultrasound should adjust your due date is if there is a big (greater than 5 to 7 days) discrepancy early on in the first trimester. After the first trimester, no matter what the later ultrasound says, the original due date established by your provider **doesn't change**. Once that date is established in the first trimester and confirmed by ultrasound, the measurements obtained at the second and third trimester ultrasounds are used as an *indicator of growth*, not a revised due date or a predictor of the day you'll go into labour. The ultrasound measurements rarely give the exact same due date as the one your provider gave you since the dates calculated on ultrasound are based purely on the size of the fetus. Normal growth is based on a bell curve, with very few people being perfectly average. There is great body diversity among the human population which is already evident very early on in the development of the fetus.

Let's say your due date is Jan. 10, and you are attending your 20 week scan. Ultrasound measurements are done and you are excited to see that the dates coming up on the machine say Jan. 5. This doesn't mean your due date needs to be revised or that you are going to give birth early! It only means that the fetus is growing at a slightly better-than-average rate. At 20 weeks, **normal** ranges of growth can be approximately 12–15 days ahead of, or behind, the due date.

Another common scenario: you are in the third trimester at 32 weeks, due on Jan. 10, but the ultrasound now says Dec. 28. It can be exciting to think that the baby may come earlier, but the fact is that it will still be 40 weeks old or

RULE OF THUMB: Due date = 40 weeks + 0 days gestation. Due date does **not** predict the day you will go into labour. Only 5% of babies are actually born on their due date. While your provider doesn't necessarily expect you to give birth that day, establishing a due date is not a futile exercise. It lets your provider know when it's the proper time to perform the various tests which need to be done at specific times in the pregnancy. It also helps them decide how far beyond your due date you should safely be allowed to go before considering induction, or when it is safe to schedule a cesarean should you need one.

'due' on Jan. 15. Babies that are growing well don't necessarily come earlier just because they are big. In the third trimester, size estimates have an even larger normal range than the second trimester. Now it's a plus-or-minus of approximately 14–21 days. Even if the fetus is measuring much smaller or larger than the normal range at any of these scans, we reiterate that your official due date shouldn't be changed. Rather, if there is a discrepancy, your provider might want to do follow up scans to ensure that the growth isn't lagging or that the baby isn't going to be excessively large towards term. It can be very hard to get patients to accept that just because the baby looks big on ultrasound, this does not imply that the due date moves up. Big babies don't necessarily come early, nor do their lungs mature any sooner than their smaller peers. Similarly, if measurements estimate the fetus is a size corresponding to a later due date than was already established, it doesn't mean it should stay 'in' longer. In fact, quite the opposite may be true. If the fetus truly is growing poorly, it might not be getting the oxygen and nutrients it requires and might need an early birth.

'Should I bring siblings to see the ultrasound?' This can be a difficult decision, with no right or wrong answer. Some facilities will clearly request that children not be brought into the exam room. They can be distracting, and there is always the possibility that they could be disruptive, get hurt, or damage equipment. If your facility allows it, parents need to make an informed decision about bringing children in to see the scan *in advance*, to avoid unpleasant situations. Parents often want to bring siblings to see and bond with their new brother or sister, and in many cases it can be a lot of fun, especially if the child or children are old enough to understand what is happening. However, in many providers' experience, young children simply don't understand that the black and white images on the screen represent their future sibling. They get hyped up in the waiting room, told to be patient, and told 'you're going to get to see the baby.' They then go to a dark room and see a strange picture on the screen that doesn't look like any baby they've ever seen. Even older children (and adults too!) sometimes don't understand what they're seeing, and while they may find it interesting for a short while, they often lose interest. The scans can take a long time to complete, especially the 20 week anatomy scan, so it is important to consider your child's attention span and ability to happily stay in a darkened room for half an hour or more. The early scans will be quicker, but might be transvaginal, limiting your access to your child, their toys, etc. Additionally, the vaginal scan may prompt uncomfortable questions about what's happening to mother under the sheet. In addition, some children are already (even unknowingly) jealous of the attention being paid to this 'other baby,' and choose this moment to demand some attention for themselves. Some mothers become upset because their child or children won't let them enjoy or even watch the images on the screen.

In other instances, some children become terrified or threatened that some-one they don't trust in medical clothes or a lab coat is doing something to their mother, and they become hysterical. In some instance, the provider has to abandon efforts and reschedule the scan altogether. Having a spouse and/or grandparent or friend there who is willing to take the child (or children) out of the room if they get too bored or upset is a really good idea. However, even with a spouse there to help keep watch, little ones can run wild, turn off the computer, try to play with the sharps (needles) disposal bin, reach into the garbage filled with nasty medical waste, and so forth.

An important note: If you know that your child has a preference for having a brother or a sister and you plan to find out the sex, we would strongly cau-tion you to either **not** bring them to see the scan, or to arrange for the sonog-rapher to keep the gender quiet until after the child is out of earshot. Countless times, children have dissolved into serious tears because the baby isn't what they want. Obviously, they are going to get this news eventually, but the ultra-sound room is not the right place, while parents are trying to watch and bond with their unborn baby and the sonographer is working hard trying to verify that the fetus has all the appropriate parts and is healthy. This raises one final point regarding siblings in the room: there is always the possibility, especially during the first trimester, that there might be a problem with the pregnancy. Having other children there can make a tough situation even harder.

Despite all that we've mentioned, people bring children to see the scans every day, and most of the time it is fine. You and your children are likely to enjoy the experience if you plan ahead and take into account your child's age and temperament, bring some distractions, and, most importantly, another adult to help if the child has had enough. However, first check the policy of the facil-ity where you are going to have your sonograms, since some facilities may have specific rules or restrictions.

Appendix

Additional websites

For further information, the following websites may be helpful. Although these are reputable sites, we cannot guarantee the accuracy of the information they contain.

General information: The following sites contain some good information about many of the more common questions during pregnancy, including general medical information, pregnancy calendars, web chats, and product recommendations/advertising.

- www.babycentre.co.uk/pregnancy

- www.babycenter.com/pregnancy

- www.babycare.co.uk

- www.pregnancy.about.com

- www.pregnancy.more4kids.info

General medical-based information and forums:

- www.webmd.com/baby

- www.patient.co.uk

- www.medhelp.org

- www.mayoclinic.com

Non-directive support and information for parents throughout the antenatal testing process, excellent resource if testing results are abnormal:

- www.arc-uk.org

Information on twins/multiples:

* www.multiples.about.com

* www.twinsonline.org.uk

Medical information and support for Trisomy 13/18, and related chromosomal disorders:

* www.soft.org.uk

* www.trisomy.org

Information and support for families and people with Down's Syndrome:

* www.downsyndrome.com

* www.downs-syndrome.org.uk

Index